THE CULTURE OF CARE IN BRITAIN SINCE THE SECOND WORLD WAR

Bernice Martin

BRISTOL
UNIVERSITY
PRESS

First published in Great Britain in 2025 by

Bristol University Press
University of Bristol
1–9 Old Park Hill
Bristol
BS2 8BB
UK
t: +44 (0)117 374 6645
e: bup-info@bristol.ac.uk

Details of international sales and distribution partners are available at bristoluniversitypress.co.uk

British Library Cataloguing in Publication Data
A catalogue record for this book is available from the British Library

ISBN 978-1-5292-4817-3 hardcover
ISBN 978-1-5292-4818-0 ePub
ISBN 978-1-5292-4819-7 ePdf

Cover design: Qube Design
Front cover image: Stocksy/Clive Watts
Bristol University Press uses environmentally responsible print partners.
Printed and bound in Great Britain by CPI Group (UK) Ltd, Croydon, CR0 4YY

FSC
www.fsc.org
MIX
Paper | Supporting responsible forestry
FSC® C013604

In memory of David

For Izaak, of course, Jonathan, Jessica,
Magnus and all their families

Contents

About the Author

Bernice Martin is Emeritus Reader in Sociology at Royal Holloway, University of London. She taught Sociology in Bedford College and then Royal Holloway College from 1961 to 1988. She taught in America at Southern Methodist University, Dallas, and had a research attachment at Boston University for parts of the 1980s and 1990s when she took part with her husband, David Martin, in research on Pentecostalism in Latin America.

Acknowledgements

During the isolation of lockdown in 2020 my son Izaak suggested I should write about care. He persuaded me to watch Ken Loach films with him and gave me a book of Tony Walsh's poetry. The book I subsequently wrote is probably not quite what he hoped for – academic habits die hard and I found myself pursuing unfinished intellectual business of my own. But this book is offered as a tribute to him, not just for his faithful work in the care sector but for the fortitude, gallantry and humour with which he has faced the many adversities which life has thrown his way.

I owe thanks to many other members of my family. Jessica and Francis read the whole manuscript and enriched me with innumerable conversations on this and many subjects, with hospitality, books, references and unstinting encouragement. Jonathan read the finished draft and gave me valued assessments and generous encouragement. My youngest sister, Gwynneth, urged me on, supplied me with new details of our family history, found old copies of the 'prize' books for me in charity shops and is a continual inspiration to me.

My intellectual debts are numerous, not least to the many scholars whose work I use in the book. Above all, I owe a fundamental intellectual debt to my late husband. Yet the problems of care that engage me in this book very seldom featured in our conversation sustained over nearly sixty years and I cannot guess what David would have made of my argument here.

I owe much to former colleagues, especially Hilary Land. I thank Grace Davie for reading the first draft so sympathetically, providing amplifications and additional references and for suggesting I should send it to Bristol University Press. The three referees to whom the Press sent the manuscript (they know who they are) provided constructive comments and additional references. I thank them all and apologize that the word limit prevented me from responding as fully as I should have liked.

I heartily thank my editors at Bristol University Press for their patience with the deficiencies of my computer skills.

1

Introduction: Apologia and Recollection

It was probably at the end of 1968 when the middle two of our four children were five and three years old that they invented a game they called 'I couldn't care less!' Their Montessori preschool took them to a pantomime that turned out to be a Moral Re-Armament Christmas show – *Give a Dog a Bone* (dir Cass 1964). It ran for years during the pantomime season at the Westminster Theatre in London, and in 1965 had become a commercial film (also directed by Cass). I never discovered the plot, because the children never felt it mattered enough to tell me. What they took from the play was the raucous game they played all over the house and garden. They were being rats. In the play whenever a child said 'I couldn't care less!', he or she turned into a rat. The children obviously thought the rats had the best time. My daughter thinks the actors who played the rats were probably acrobatic dancers, because they tumbled and leapt excitingly about the stage. Her little brother, who was already the comic of the family, revelled in shouting 'I couldn't care less!', grinning broadly, dancing wildly, throwing his arms around, pulling comical faces and turning somersaults.

I have thought a lot about this game and its tag line in the last few years as I have worried about the inadequate funding of the care sector of the welfare state and the burdens of care, paid and unpaid, that fall so disproportionately on poor women and not a few poor men, many of them from ethnic minority or immigrant sectors of our population. These worries have been sharpened in recent years by witnessing the strain on the NHS and the health and social care system at close quarters during that same son's year-long illness in 2014 and slow, very partial recuperation from encephalitis, which left him disabled and unable to work, and again during the months of my husband's final illness before he died at home in 2019 in the care of the family, the wonderful community nurses of the local hospice and the frantically overworked continuing care teams of two private companies franchised through social care, one of them almost exclusively staffed by

Ugandan migrants. Even before the COVID-19 pandemic struck, I had begun to wonder about what has happened to the culture of caring over the course of my lifetime, but my sense of urgency was heightened by the emergency and how we responded to it. There was unfailing selfless care by front-line staff, again with people who were at the time labelled BAME (Black, Asian and minority ethnic) workers heavily over-represented among them, and after the first ruthless assault on the supermarkets to stockpile groceries, an upsurge of volunteers emerged to help others and there seemed to be a selective recovery of neighbourliness. But the ever-widening health inequalities, the woeful inadequacy of the funding, even more so of social care than of the health sector, have also been fully exposed by the pandemic. The public even felt impelled to raise money as well as offer volunteer labour for what is not a charity but a state-provided service funded by our taxes. The shocking inequalities in Britain have been brutally exposed in the skewed distribution of deaths from the virus, again hitting the poor, the vulnerable and ethnic minority populations hardest.

We have been left in no doubt just how low caring comes in the hierarchy of the state's routine economic priorities – outside a sudden emergency that involves us all – and how much caring is defined as 'unskilled' or even not 'work' at all when provided by the family. The COVID-19 epidemic threw our cultural and moral priorities into turmoil as economic and political imperatives faced off against the moral imperative of preserving lives, especially the lives of the vulnerable, dependent and weak – the 'unproductive' – most of whom, fortunately, still have votes. As we emerged from the emergency, the usual economic priorities and ways of thinking reasserted themselves with renewed force in a period of rising cost of living and government-incurred debt from the pandemic, on top of the long austerity politically imposed in the wake of the 2007–08 financial crisis, which itself accelerated the increasing inequality of wealth and income distribution among us. The heroism of the carers has been rewarded by token gestures rather than by a radical rethink of the patterns of remuneration and a revision of the low value we routinely place on all those 'unskilled' caring tasks. Instead we face recurrent threats of economic stagnation or even recession, with national strategies, after Brexit, that redouble the power of capitalist economic values and ethnocentric political priorities.

The pungent irony of my children's game was always obvious. I realized that the moral of the performance in the theatre could only have been the importance of caring for others. The son who got so much fun from the game of 'I couldn't care less!' had been born with a genetic abnormality, Noonan syndrome, which, among other things, severely restricted his height and made him vulnerable to lung infections and heart problems. As an adult, he was a committed care worker for two decades and more. When encephalitis struck him, he was a driver/carer of adults with severe learning difficulties and other serious physical and mental health problems. He was and is fiercely protective of the rights and dignity of the disabled, the 'different' and the 'useless', and is morally and politically opposed to policies that might 'solve' the problem by eliminating it – for example, by routinely recommending abortion. He now finds himself trapped in distressing social 'uselessness' by fear that if he embarks on any volunteering within his capacities, he might lose his Personal Independence Payment and Employment and Support Allowance because it could be construed as evidence of his ability to work. As I write this in late summer 2023, he is currently fearful about initiatives proposed by the Conservative government to 'encourage' people on disablement benefits back into work. His older sister is a priest who spends a good deal of time, as most of her clerical colleagues do, bringing care and dignity to the dying, the bereaved, the lonely, the disturbed, and very often to the 'difficult' who turn to the clergy when they have worn out the available care the mental health and social care system, and sometimes even their own families, can give them.

I can't believe that the Moral Re-Armament message of *Give a Dog a Bone* fundamentally shaped either of the children: their commitment to caring for others began in their childhood care for each other. Their elder brother has worked for most of his working life with the homeless and vulnerable and latterly for a charity, and none of the four has ever valued wealth or a large income as any kind of priority in life. Although the youngest of the four is a rock musician, he is emphatically not one of the super-rich but someone who opted for the 'alternative society' after university because he believed it was a place where 'people take care of each other "off grid"'. Maybe some of the altruistic messages of the counterculture got through to all four of them – certainly our youngest son, who was born in 1971, never stops wishing he had been born sooner so that he could have been part of its golden age that spanned his brothers' and sister's formative years. In some respects, the altruism of the counterculture was often a secular (or 'spiritual' or 'pagan') transmutation of Christian cultural values of care for others. Even so, the counterculture played its own part in eroding the culture of care that I knew in my own formative years. My analysis of what I think that culture was, and what transformed it, includes the paradoxical collusion between, on the one hand, aspects of the counterculture and the 'alternative society' and, on the other, the atomistic individualism that fuels the excesses of 'consumer society' and neoliberal capitalism and has done so much to shape the hedonistic imagination of what Olivier Roy calls 'the culture of the desiring self' (Roy 2019, 2020).

What I argue in this book inevitably will be inflected by the position and values from which the author writes, so this first chapter is an attempt to situate the perspective that grew from my own experience, observations and judgements, even though such attempts are inescapably partial and blinkered. I write as a professional sociologist but what follows will be as much what my late husband, a sociologist, theologian and priest, called 'thinking with your life' as it is formal sociology (Martin 2018). I do not have the background in social policy that would enable me to dissect the welfare policies that got us to this pass, but I have spent my professional life analysing cultural and religious change. I begin therefore from my own location in this cultural history of care, starting with the problems thrown up for me by educational mobility and my Christian background and the intersection of both with the dramatic feminism of the 1970s and its sharp critique of gendered caring.

My generation came just before the baby boomers, neither firmly prewar – I was born in 1937 – nor postwar. Our childhood was dominated by the war years and the austerity that followed, with youth and, in my case, higher education arriving just as the mid-1950s began to offer glimpses of less straitened possibilities. I was part of an early cohort of working-class scholarship children who were offered postwar educational mobility when it was still very restricted. When I was a student, the cohort of state-funded veterans of the war had already graduated – two of my university teachers were among them. The university sector covered 4 per cent of my age cohort, and of that tiny minority, less than one-fifth of women undergraduates came from a class background like mine and perhaps up to a quarter of the men, while the manual working class still made up over two-thirds of the population. Most of the women graduates from a semi-skilled working-class family like mine became schoolteachers, while their brothers became engineers, teachers or occasionally went into the civil service or business (Mandler 2020, p 88; De Bellaigue et al 2022; Blackburn and Jarman 1993). By the time of the baby boomer generation, those born between the mid-1940s and the mid-1960s, the range of employment had expanded, opening far more options to them, including new white-collar and professional work. That expansion and differentiation of the economy, even more than the postwar drive to increase educational opportunity, was what made possible the rising social mobility of the baby boomers and gave that generation and the one after the misleading impression that life could only go on getting better for everyone, at least in terms of jobs and incomes. The baby boomers, which include several of my six younger siblings, found openings in advertising, sales, banking, market research, insurance, business, retail, laboratory work, pharmacy work and social work or in an ever-expanding leisure sector and many other new areas of the economy as well as the developing public service sectors of the welfare state and the nationalized utilities. That generation created and consumed postwar youth culture and largely founded the 'popular' sector of what are now called the 'creative industries', which today are a significant segment of the British economy.

I and my university contemporaries were at the beginning of our thirties and most of us were already established in our adult families and our professions when the new feminism began to make waves, roughly from 1970 after the protests at the Miss World contest at the Albert Hall that year caused a media furore. The international bestsellers *The Female Eunuch* by Germaine Greer and *Sexual Politics* by Kate Millett both appeared in that same year (Greer 1970; Millett 1970). By this time I was married and responsible for a teenage stepson and two school-age children as well as holding a full-time academic post. I had been well schooled in the suffragist principles of the first generation of women graduates, some of whom taught at my girls' grammar school, all unmarried and many of them very accomplished scholars. Like them, I fervently believed in women's education and our right to fulfilling work. I knew, for example, that my distinguished headmistress had earned her university education by becoming a 'normal school'[1] teacher, which then gained her a place to read classics in her local northern redbrick university. There, her brilliant first class degree enabled her to go on to an equally distinguished Doctorate of Divinity. I knew too that my inspiring English teacher, who produced the school's biennial Shakespeare play, had been one of the early Cambridge women students originally denied graduation however brilliantly they had performed in the final examinations. I understood that education was something admirable women thrived on and my university education in a women's college reinforced the message.

I identified in principle with the feminist movement, but there were aspects of the militant new wave of the late 1960s and 1970s that made me uneasy in ways I shall explore more fully in due course. Most of my disquiet concerned class, caring and (already unfashionably) religion. Many of the stars among the new young feminists seemed to have middle-class or even more privileged backgrounds, and the assumptions they brought with them were very different from mine. In the department where I taught sociology, the most militant feminist and political radical in the late 1960s was a woman economist from Oxford who had been one of the last batch of debutants to be presented at court in 1958 (O'Driscoll 2022). She inspired her students with Marxist anti-colonial views about capitalism as well as radical feminist ideas. At the beginning of the 1970s, shortly after she left the college, she joined the Provisional IRA and took part in some of its operations (O'Driscoll 2022).[2] She was, of course, exceptional among the committed feminists I knew, but for the rest, what I found particularly troubling at the time was not so much their political radicalism as their attacks, including from some Christian feminists, on the 'reactionary', 'patriarchal' assumption that women were and should be carers. I had a queasy feeling that rhetoric condemning caring as intrinsically demeaning to women was in danger of rubbishing my mother and all my women forbears, whose hard lives had been spent doing just that, often while working in the cotton mill as well. And it was not as if their menfolk had had an easy time of it as manual workers doing long hours in exhausting and often dirty jobs. I also believed in caring for others, one's neighbour as well as one's own, as a core value of the Christian faith – the inclusion of this belief is the reason why the newly fashionable ideas of Friedrich Nietzsche condemned Christianity as a religion only fit for slaves. Yet when I was eight years old, at the end of the war, my notions of who needed our – my – care were shocked and irreversibly expanded by the pictures and news items of the liberation of the Nazi concentration camps. I studied sociology in university out of a Christian conviction that had universalized my idea of who my neighbour was and in the ignorant supposition that the discipline might show me how society's care for the least fortunate, including the people I grew up with in the North West of England, could be made fairer.

I soon learned not only that much of sociology had a secularist programme, either explicitly or implicitly, but also that it elaborated problems of social injustice and inequality more readily than the always equivocal solutions, with the disheartening 'unintended consequences'. Nevertheless, the discipline overall maintained an optimistic or even crusading spirit of 'progress'. In the early 1970s, I still harboured a residue of the naive optimism imbibed with the theories, as distinct from the actual findings, of sociology and had not yet wholly jettisoned a blind confidence in the intrinsic goodness of human beings and the possibility of straightforwardly living according to Christian principles. Life, and academic politics (which I was slow to realize did not show the incorruptible integrity that I had come to expect from the example of my headmistress), painfully taught me the potency and ubiquity of realpolitik at every level. My own costly achievement of a realistic rather than a stubbornly optimistic hope for sociology, the Christian faith and the species *Homo sapiens* is another story that need not concern us here except to note that I had barely begun to work through its knots when I found myself having to react to the 1970s surge of feminist protest. I did so with a troubling ambivalence that came from my class background and my Christian convictions, at a time of upheavals and challenges from the counterculture and several varieties of political radicalism on university campuses and in the wider political world.

I was the eldest of seven children in a working-class family. The cotton town where we lived was Lowry country. Its townscapes were the backdrop to what Anne M. Wagner in her essay on Lowry calls 'the social geography of working-class experience' (Wagner 2013, p 77). Shirley Baker's photographs of Manchester and Salford at the start of the 1960s slum clearance give an accurate and eloquent picture of the streets I remember from the 1940s – damp, decaying terraced houses with outside lavatories and no domestic amenities; although our houses were smaller than the once grander terraces of the central city that she photographed in their terminal agony (Baker 2018).[3] I have a particularly strong recollection of my mother's never-ending war against decay and the damp that oozed from the rotting window frames and windowsills whatever heroic efforts she made.

My childhood had left me in no doubt about the pivotal importance of women and with an unshakeable conviction that women could do anything they put their minds to, which was perhaps one reason I had embarked so confidently on combining marriage and a ready-made family with a demanding job. I was additionally buoyed by my husband's belief that there was nothing women could not or should not do (including all the traditionally male chores that he found so impossible himself and that his omnicompetent mother had taken in her stride). In my childhood, there had been very few adult males around until 1945–46, apart from a few older uncles whose own war had been in 1914–18. All the able-bodied men, including my father and some of my much older cousins, had gone away to the war. Women did everything, and families were heavily dependent on mothers, grandmothers, sisters and women neighbours, whose mutual help and ingenuity in managing tiny incomes and widespread shortages made the difference between abject poverty and something marginally better.

My mother and her eight sisters (some of the older ones had children who were around my mother's age), although they were prone to little 'feuds', operated as a quasi-collective, helping each other out without question when funds were especially tight, handing on children's clothes, sharing food and always stepping in during the 'lying in' period after a birth, when new mothers at that time had to stay in bed and needed help with any toddlers and older children. I and my second brother acquired 'second homes' with one of our older aunts, starting when we had each been whisked off as toddlers at the birth of the next baby. My mother and women like her positively welcomed rationing, which at least meant they were guaranteed the basics to feed their families. It was some years before I recognized that my mother's preference for dry biscuits with a scrape of margarine as her meal – Mum's eternal Ryvitas were a standing joke – had been her way of making sure the rest of us had enough to eat. All that changed remarkably little in that first decade after the war, when my father and the other men were back in their jobs again. The intelligent 'managing' by women like my mother and the mutual support of the women's networks remained vital even in the 1950s period of full employment and then especially when the cotton industry began to run into postwar competition from abroad and my father was sometimes working three-day weeks.

When I went to university shortly after my father's sudden death at the age of 42, my relatives and neighbours left me in no doubt about my mother's sacrificial heroism, not to say foolishness, in letting me take up my scholarship when my next younger brother, just starting his apprenticeship, was 'going out to work to keep her'. My mother was now a widow with seven dependent children, the youngest not yet two years old, and she was 'making ends meet' on a widow's pension by taking care of all the neighbours' children while their mothers were at work. All of us got Saturday jobs as soon as we were old enough, and I offered to abandon university but my mother would not hear of it. She thought that would betray my father's dearest wish: he had been embarrassingly proud when news of my state scholarship was published in the local paper on the morning of his fatal heart attack.

I went to university with a mixture of exhilaration and guilt, and had recurrent nightmares about not being at home to protect my younger brothers and sisters or contribute to the family income. I spent as little money as possible and sent much of my grant to my mother. The first Christmas vacation back home, I realized how agitated my mother had been in case I had grown apart from the family and didn't want to come home, even though I had sent her long letters every week. I knew that her own mother had not allowed her clever daughter (penultimate child of nine girls and one surviving boy) to take up her scholarship to the local authority secondary school. My grandmother had not even allowed my mother to apply for shop or office work when she left the church elementary school at 14 in 1928. Her schooling had ended abruptly when the school was closed early for the summer because of a smallpox outbreak. My mother remembered being 'clouted round the head' by Grandma in the employment exchange on the Friday afternoon when she left school, for getting above herself when she had suggested a job that would let her wear shoes instead of clogs. She had to go into the mill, the same as her sisters, 'and like it'. No summer holiday, but the very next Monday morning straight to the bleaching and dying works with her brother. There, she met my father, her brother's friend.

As a sociology student, I had been taught Talcott Parsons' early argument that social mobility inevitably separates the nuclear family from the extended family, partly because the rivalry between fathers and sons requires a socially mobile son's family to be free of obligations to kin, in particular not to be subordinated to the authority of his lower-status father.[4] I heard something very like it, again attributed to Parsons, from American sociologist Peter Berger, pronounced almost as a moral principle, when my husband and I spent some time at Boston University in the 1990s, working with Peter and renting the apartment at the top of his house. Peter was incredulous that I had invited my mother and a couple of my siblings and their families to stay with us for a spring holiday. The Parsons argument he quoted at me then, in something between a joke and a complaint, had surfaced earlier in relation to the research on Pentecostals in Latin America in which we were engaged, with the added refinement that releasing the nuclear family from wider kinship obligations makes it easier for Pentecostals to distance themselves from pre-Christian ancestor rituals and, the clincher for Peter, frees them to follow new entrepreneurial possibilities.

Yet, a few years earlier, my husband and I had taken my mother with us, not from Boston but from Dallas, on a research weekend in Mexico, where our driver took us to meet his extended family. They were several households all living in a small suburban enclave of smart houses with everyone assembled in the matriarch's kitchen at the end of the day. My mother had delighted the Mexicans with her spontaneous exclamation on meeting them: 'How marvellous! You have *real* families like us!' These Mexicans were an educationally mobile, four-generation Pentecostal family that included Bible translators and doctors. Our young driver was the one renegade who had discovered the bohemian life, initially through the poems of Baudelaire. He had come right out of his family's religious culture and their hard-won bourgeois achievement into a secular life of self-expression and financial insecurity, which made him very dependent on his kin for intermittent support, including housing. But this was not the 'anecdotal evidence' with which to parry Peter Berger's settled conviction about the impossibility of extended families in mobile modernity.

The social mobility of daughters did not get much attention from Parsons or anyone else in my undergraduate sociology classes in the 1950s or for some time after that, but even as a student with everything still to learn I was always awkwardly conscious of a disjunction between the theory and my own experience. The postwar social mobility research in British sociology was for a long time entirely concentrated on males, while popular novels and films in the 1950s and early 1960s were full of rebellious working-class 'angry young men' desperate to escape the constraints of family, respectability and commitments of any sort. A review of the 2021 memoir of David Storey, rugby professional turned novelist and playwright, from a Yorkshire miner's family, has recently repeated those familiar tropes about the struggles and alienation of socially and culturally mobile men in the 1950s through Storey's sense that his cultural activities were not 'real work' like going down the pit (Storey 2021; Taylor 2021). Social mobility among women has received scant attention by comparison, particularly the way in which for some of us it is not so much our father's paid work as our mother's taken-for-granted caring and thankless household drudgery that is the 'real' work, while scholarship or writing can feel like a selfish and unjustified indulgence, as David Storey sometimes felt about the comparative validity of writing plays and hewing coal. The unacknowledged assumption about gender differences was one reason why, for instance, it took sociologists of education right up to the 1990s to recognize that sampling error was not the reason behind repeated findings showing African Caribbean girls educationally outperforming not only their male counterparts but, on average, both males and females of similar class origins in the White British population. Female educational mobility is *not* the same as it is for their male class or ethnic peers: it can have quite different social meanings for young women. They may anticipate life as primary 'breadwinner' and/or anchor of an extended family, as many Black British girls did in the 1990s, and as some still do.

The feminist historian Carolyn Steedman has a different narrative of educational mobility for girls in her brilliant meditation on her own conflicted childhood, *Landscape for a Good Woman* (Steedman 1986). She describes school, books and, later, university as her defence and escape from the home life that left her both hating and mirroring her dissatisfied and frustrated mother. She describes the significant context of her own early years as 'a Lancashire childhood', the working-class family background that her mother carried within her when she fled to London looking for a better life. The unsatisfying (and unconsecrated) relationship with Steedman's father did not provide it, and she effectively sidelined him from the family. Like Steedman's mother, mine was 'a good mother', a badge of honour given not by herself – at least not explicitly as Steedman's mother did – but by neighbours and relatives. I never doubted it and internalized it without the kind of conflict and resistance that Steedman suffered, even as I reached for an altogether more expansive existence with my father's active encouragement.

In the early 1980s, the American feminist psychologist Carol Gilligan was instrumental in transforming a number of paradigms in the social sciences and in ethical thinking about caring. Gilligan's research demonstrated that the pattern of women and girls routinely prioritizing human connection and interdependence over individual competitiveness is foundational to female moral development (Gilligan 1982). This underlies findings on the educational mobility of Caribbean British girls and a number of related issues as well as my own response to educational mobility and my chronic urge to defuse potential conflicts rather than let them rip. But it also raises the question of how far this pattern is a specific historical product rather than an essential, ahistorical and acultural female characteristic. Gilligan has recently published a new assessment of her four decades of research on the way young boys and girls learn how to ignore and suppress what they really know (Gilligan 2023).That 'other' (unacknowledged) voice can only be detected in the contradictions that slip out in interviews, only for the interviewee to swiftly silence them. Gilligan sees this as a self-inflicted injury, inflicted in the interest of becoming 'men' and 'women' who will be acceptable to others in a society structured by patriarchy. She draws out its implications for the ethic of care for others and extends its relevance to men as well as women: caring is everyone's proper business. Her case is that this 'moral injury' that little boys and rather older girls suffer results in a sexual binary that makes females value care and connection and cuts males off from both. Whatever aspects of cultural 'masculinity' in the form of individualism and competitiveness were required from me in order to be educationally successful, I was self-consciously unwilling to allow them to demand radical detachment from my family and class or upend my conviction that the moral priority of care for others is unnegotiable.

As a student, I was desperate not to betray my family and was binding myself close to it even as my own life diverged into very different cultural territory, markedly distinct from that of my clever working-class brothers. That divergence, and my determination not to let it estrange me from the family, began at school, particularly after I won a scholarship to the local direct grant girls' grammar school. My mother feared we would not be able to afford the uniform, just as in her own schooldays her mother had. My mother worried, even then, that if I went to the grammar school, I might decide the family was not good enough for me. My father, who normally left all decisions to my mother, on this matter insisted I should not miss my chance. After all, though boys needed 'a good trade', girls could become teachers. His manager in the bleaching and dyeing works, who was paying fees to send his only son to the parallel boys' grammar school, thought it would be a shame not to let me take up a coveted free place. This same manager, during my O Level year, took me to my first live orchestral concert, which included a performance of Shostakovich's Fifth Symphony by the Hallé Orchestra that I found so powerful that I have never forgotten the occasion or lost my love for Shostakovich's music.

My father's family was small – he was the youngest of three boys – and his next older brother, 'our kid', had been a conscientious objector in the war and became a mental health nurse following his alternative war service. Uncle Charlie had what my mother mocked as pretentions and even owned a few popular operatic records. Their mother had been 'in service' and a widow since 1918. She took in army officers as lodgers during the Second World War. She and my mother did not get on, especially as during the war my grandmother seldom encouraged visits from me and my brothers in case we disturbed 'her' officers. To my mother, her mother-in-law was a 'snob' with no good reason – 'all swank'. I didn't realize it at the time, but my father's eldest brother, 'little Walter', had been born illegitimately to an unknown, or at least never acknowledged, father seven years before my grandmother and grandfather married in 1909. When my youngest sister recently traced the family tree, she found that in 1906, four years after Walter was born in a mother and baby home, not in my grandmother's home area of Herefordshire but in Greater Manchester, Grandma had been admitted to a workhouse (by Emmeline Pankhurst herself, the Registrar for Manchester) and had lived there with the boy for a year. A further illegitimate son had been born after she left to try to support herself and her sons. They were obliged to return to the workhouse and the malnourished baby stayed there when Grandma left with Walter, but died a few weeks later and was buried in an unmarked workhouse plot. Knowing fragments of this story may have been at the root of my mother's resentment of her mother-in-law's social snobbery. It does much to explain Grandma T's determination to cling to any tokens of gentility that had rubbed off from her employers and 'her' officers. As a child, I knew nothing of it, and I very much doubt that my mother knew about the baby who died in the workhouse.

During my grammar school years, I tried to introduce my family to all the exciting new things that were being unfolded to me, but apart from my father, who responded especially to the classical music I was discovering, I found them pretty resistant. To my younger brothers, it was all sissy stuff, all right for a girl but lethal for a boy's reputation with his friends. They stuck to maths and sciences and the new youth culture, starting with skiffle and later rock and mod styles. My closest brother, two years younger than me, only recently told our youngest sister how he had learned not to do too well at his secondary modern school after the first time he was praised by the French teacher for his pronunciation. He got so much ribbing from his footballing mates that he always pronounced French words, and everything else, with an aggressively Lancashire accent after that. He carefully contrived to do badly in his exams, not so badly as to worry our parents but badly enough not to provoke the scorn of his friends. He went into an apprenticeship after school and became a meticulous and highly skilled carpenter who reads science books for pleasure and still plays walking football in his eighties. He was my mother's mainstay after my father died and I went away to university.

All my brothers were horrified by the amount of homework I got from school and preferred 'playing out' with their friends in the street or the park. Shirley Baker's photographs show just such gangs of northern children at their street games. My brothers never understood why I liked doing the homework, just as I enjoyed going to school and to church and Sunday school. The parish church at the centre of the town where we were sent by our parents every Sunday was the place where I first discovered the sensibility that thrived in the grammar school and was fed by the BBC, particularly through *Children's Hour*. I came to love the Book of Common Prayer, the language, the ritual, the music, Bach preludes and fugues on the organ, the congregational Anglican chant to the Psalms. The choir (all male, of course) sang early contrapuntal settings of the service or anthems and canticles by Byrd, Weelkes or Tallis, Parry or Howells that sometimes raised goosebumps as I listened. But the reluctant train of little brothers I had to take to Sunday school couldn't wait to be old enough to get out of it all, as all the men in the family did. Apart from the two who married Roman Catholics, my mother's many sisters were assiduous churchgoers, mostly regulars at the eight o'clock Communion service, and active members of the Mothers' Union, but their 'heathen' husbands never entered church except for christenings, weddings and funerals. My father had been sent to Methodist Sunday school but never went to church once he started work. Something must have stuck from that Methodist background, because, like my teetotal maternal grandfather, he was 'not much of a drinker', which made all the difference to the family finances. Like most of my uncles, my father was a devoted member of his trade union and member of a mutual society. Some of my older aunts and uncles were Labour Party members. I ran as the class candidate for Labour in the 1951 election in my grammar school and, as I had expected, lost heavily to the Conservative candidate, even though I knew we had the better case. I bored my poor family with my political hectoring for years.

When an eccentric friend from school (hers was one of a few Labour families among the 'scholarship girls' at school) insisted on bringing her cello to our house, my brothers howled like ghosts through the chimney as she played, though she barely noticed. All through school, I was wracked by the sense that my success at school and my delight in what was championed, and later denigrated, as 'high culture' was the very thing that was building an insuperable barrier preventing my brothers from having any curiosity about it, let alone exploring it. They were all successful in different ways. One moved from the technical school to an engineering apprenticeship that led into an engineering degree and then to building power stations all over the world. The two who went to the local authority grammar school left school at 16 after good O Levels; one became a senior manager of an insurance company, valued for his early expertise in computers, and the other became the youngest dealer on the Manchester stock exchange. My middle sister became a smart receptionist. With the exception of the engineer, none of them ever regretted staying in the place where they were born or not developing a passion for literature and classical music; and they all gave church a wide berth. My youngest sister, born when I was 17, was the exception, though she has never been a churchgoer as an adult and did not settle away from the town where we were brought up. She started working in local authority residential children's homes and eventually became a child protection social worker, picking up two degrees in the process; she developed her own taste for modern literature, theatre, film and art. She is a Labour voter and a convinced feminist, though far from rejecting caring for others, which was anyway the rationale of her demanding profession. She is no sentimentalist but a realist who does her best to encourage people to become independent rather than inviting their dependence on her or others. She also acts as the historian and anchor of the extended family; this starts with her own children and includes a small tribe of cousins as well as our siblings and their families. She and I never lived in the same household after I left for university when she was a toddler, and her contemporary tastes are entirely her own doing and almost as exotic to our siblings as mine are.

My ambivalent response to the feminism of the 1970s was refracted through that family and class experience and my acute appreciation of the intelligence that my mother and women like her had needed to keep their families fed, clothed and flourishing in hard times, both during the war and in the years of austerity that followed it. It did certainly demand a degree of selflessness, but that seldom looked like 'playing the martyr'. They did not look to me like the caricatures of submissive ciphers of a patriarchal system that I later heard castigated, and they were far too robust and humorous to be the 'angels in the house' detested by Virginia Woolf. The women in the working classes whom I knew needed all the intelligence, resilience and toughness they could muster. The wives of the miners during the miners' strike of 1984 may have lived in families where there was more obvious male dominance than in the cotton districts, but they displayed the same strength and family loyalty that I observed in the women of my childhood.

Lancashire women managed the family purse, which was why being regarded as 'a good manager', like my mother, was the highest possible praise. The men handed over their pay packets on Friday to their mothers and later their wives, and they received their 'spending money' in return. The women, needless to say, never had spending money of their own. My mother and her sisters told stories of how their mother had acted as informal banker and sometimes physical protector for neighbours whose husbands spent their wages in the pub or gambling and left them to face the rent collector, the bailiffs and other debt enforcers. Grandma would lend the 'best clothes' of her working daughters between Monday and Friday for pawning to cover the shortfall in her women neighbours' rent and food bills, on the understanding that the clothes would be returned in time for the weekend. The only time she was found out was when the engagement ring of one of my mother's older sisters was not returned on time, and that led to an almighty row, remembered and laughed about for many years in the family. Grandma was also never found out by her older daughters for something she was afraid they might see as wasting their wages – she regularly sent my mother, as a schoolgirl, to take plates of cooked food to poorer neighbours living in elementary two-room homes of the kind my grandparents' family had rented themselves before all the girls' wages had turned them into one of the fortunate families in their street, though even then the girls had slept several to a bed. The 1911 Census, three years before my mother's birth, shows the family divided between a group of younger school-age children, toddlers and babies with one or two of the girls in work living in a two-room dwelling with their parents and another group of a few girls in work and some school-age ones living with their maternal grandmother in a nearby two-room back-to-back. The grave in the local cemetery in which this woman, my great-grandmother (daughter of an Irish father and an Italian mother from migrant communities), buried my great-grandfather after his early death also holds 17 children. Most of them were babies or infants that she and her daughters had lost (my grandmother alone lost six or seven of her children), but one seems to be the child of neighbours who probably could not afford a grave of their own. The grave papers give the identities of the occupants of the grave, but there was never enough money for a headstone so it is overgrown and hard to find among other unmarked plots and in an obscure corner. The cemetery has a plaque near the main entrance commemorating the numerous babies and young children who have no other memorial, tribute to the appalling incidence of infant mortality up to at least the 1930s among the working-class community of the area. No wonder my mother welcomed rationing, family allowances and the advent of the NHS so ardently. In 1948 she had me and my three younger brothers memorize and recite our NHS identity numbers, telling us it would always prove we were entitled to a doctor whatever happened to us.

The later relative comfort of my maternal grandparents' family was also, as my grandmother was quick to point out, the result of having married a teetotaller, 'old Methody', in 1892; he used to read his Liberal newspaper aloud on the doorstep to his less literate neighbours, and he handed over everything he earned from his two or three jobs for the family purse. Grandma controlled the entire family income from the large apron with multiple pockets that I remember her always wearing. She put all the wages into it every Friday and doled out the meagre spending money 'right up to the day before we got married', as my mother often told us. In spite of his Methodist upbringing, my father would occasionally join the other sisters' husbands in the pub on a Friday night for 'just a half' of the manly beer he really didn't like. All the men in my extended family treated their wives as 'the boss' and were gentle with their children and generous to their nephews and nieces. At the pub on those Friday nights they probably enjoyed, at the expense of the managing women, sexist jokes of the kind you could hear in the music hall and later from the comics on radio and television variety programmes. But nobody could doubt their willing dependence on those same women. (Both the brilliant Victoria Wood, who was a much younger pupil at my grammar school, and the stand-up comic, screenwriter and actor Peter Kay have mined that same deposit of Lancashire family humour today, though with a more even-handed approach to gender.) Whatever 'patriarchy' was, the term didn't really seem to apply to my uncles and father. Carolyn Steedman says something similar about her own sidelined father, but argues that it may be the surrounding society rather than a domestic patriarch that carries the information to a child about where and with whom power lies (Steedman 1986). Nowadays, anthropologists have taught us to see contradictory patterns of power and authority as evidence of 'intersectionality', constructions of layered identity that involve the distribution of different dimensions of power between genders, generations, classes, ethnicities or whatever, rather than anything so unified as unequivocal patriarchy, straightforward matriarchal power or clear evidence of 'resistance' to particular forms of dominance. But early feminism, like the sociology of that period, had not yet had the benefit of such subtleties.

Feminism in that 1970s eruption seemed paradoxical to me. As time went on, of course, it became clear that the first noisy critique of gendered caring had always been complemented by feminists who researched the unpaid work of women, including working-class women. That, to a large extent, corrected the early impression that women's caring work was *intrinsically* degrading and something every educated woman should shun. Yet the women's movement was always divided between those for whom the primary goal was the right of women to do everything men did, especially when it carried more status and significance than all the things women habitually did, and those who mainly campaigned to advance the interests of low-status and poor women. Feminist researchers and protesters for many decades demanded decent incomes for the work women did, whether it was the 'invisible' and unwaged 'reproductive work' in the family or the work in paid employment, though they seldom had immediate or spectacular political success. The postwar 'family allowance' that had proved such a salvation to my widowed mother had been introduced as part of the Beveridge policies enacted by the Labour government of 1945, but its origins go back to before the First World War in the idea, championed by Eleanor Rathbone, that women need an income for their families that they, rather than their husbands, control – not all breadwinners behaved like the ones I grew up among, but more like the husbands of my grandmother's debt-ridden neighbours. Rathbone, one of the early graduates of Somerville College, Oxford, knew the life of Liverpool dockers' families from her philanthropic work and understood that many families needed supplements to the 'breadwinner's' wages, even when they did not have men who 'drank' or gambled, simply because households contained more children than the supposed 'average' size on which a survival wage was customarily calculated.

I shall come back to some of that earlier work and also examine how class and ethnic divisions had always been a fault line in the women's movement(s). For the moment, however, I need to return to the immediate dilemmas about caring that confronted the postwar cohorts of professional women, more particularly the early quota of socially mobile women like me, in 1970 and after. Whether we were committed feminists or not, we faced a double bind: housework and caring was a necessity in any household or family but that 'second shift', as Arlie Hochschild calls it (see Hochschild and Machung 1989), did not 'count' morally or in terms of status or have any legitimate priority compared with the demands of the profession or the life of the mind. The denigration by a section of 1970s feminism of caring as part of the female gender role intensified the dilemma and sometimes made it seem to me that having children was a guilty self-indulgence that consumed time and energy stolen from more important work.

Postwar women graduates quickly learned that even when they had male partners willing and able to take their share of domestic labour and all that 'caring', the structures of work in the 'skilled' occupations and professions placed increasing demands on time and energy that made it ever harder to find what later became the mantra of 'work–life balance'. Even where partners are willing to 'help', they often find the creative aspects, such as playing with children or cooking, more palatable than the tedious repetitive labour of routine maintenance or remembering what day to put out the bins, let alone taking the responsibility for planning and organizing it all. Many married professional women found themselves faced with the problem of whether they or their husbands should go slow on their careers, since it was clear that employers increasingly required total commitment to work at the expense of any private desire or obligation. And as each generation lived longer, more women found themselves squeezed between responsibility for children at one end of their adult lives and responsibility for older family members by middle age, when their careers were at their apex and often just as children were becoming independent; the latter responsibility came about as elderly parents and grandparents were now living long enough to become infirm and need various degrees of help and care. In response, from the early 1970s professional women began to postpone marriage to a progressively later age or to avoid it altogether (marriage rates have declined year by year from a peak in 1972) and/or to postpone or even avoid childbearing (birth rates have fallen since the advent of 'the pill', especially for middle-class women, from a peak in the mid-1960s; births outside civil partnerships and marriage have spectacularly increased from less than 10 per cent in 1950 to approximately 50 per cent today; and women's age at first pregnancy has steadily risen over the same period, most notably for graduate women) (Census 2021).

Working-class families faced exactly the same problems as professional and white-collar families as increasing proportions of women joined the labour market, a trend going back to the 1950s. As families in all classes found it progressively difficult to live on one income at the standard of living which they had come to expect (the notion of *the* male breadwinner was another target of criticism for the women's movement), women recognized how hard it would be to be successful in their work or career *and* be hands-on mothers as well as doing the cleaning, washing, shopping and cooking that had to be done by someone for every household. Where there are ageing, sick or disabled family members to be cared for, the burden can be enormous. Both employers and the state continue to depend on the women in the family doing most of the invisible caring in families. Some professional women did as much of the drudgery as they and their partners could find energy and time for and recruited other women, not usually well paid or highly qualified, to replace some of that caring labour. Or, like me, they took full advantage of the 'free' services of grandparents, in my case my husband's parents, both of whom had been 'in service'. What Virginia Woolf and others in the advanced guard of professional and graduate women of the 1920s and 1930s had called 'the servant problem' had not magically gone away for us any more than it did for them, despite the arrival of all the new domestic equipment that simultaneously took over some of the most back-breaking and dirty effort and enabled ever higher standards of domestic comfort, which required yet more domestic attention. The new 'servants' might now take the form of au pairs, often from other countries or, as always, from lower-status echelons in British society, who did much of the childcare, cleaned the houses or cared for the ailing older generation, who might once have expected daughters and daughters-in-law to house and take care of them. And the new non-servants working for the new middle-class families were still almost entirely women.

The vicious circle which had poor women taking over, at very modest pay, domestic caring for highly educated professional women was not even broken for the increasing numbers of childless professionals, who still needed their cleaners and factotums. And the more these paid domestic jobs were filled by women, the harder it was to increase their rates of pay, precisely because they were doing 'women's work' and so, by definition, did not need expensive or extended training for what 'anyone could do'.

In her marvellous book *Mrs Woolf and the Servants*, Alison Light unravels the whole problem with great clarity (Light 2008). There are tasks that have to be performed in any society: caring for babies and children, caring for the bodies of people too young or too old or too infirm to do so for themselves, disposing of all the bodily debris, producing and cooking food, cleaning and maintaining living quarters, cleaning and maintaining clothing. This is *labour* – physical as well as emotional and mental. Prominent are the many manual tasks that relate intimately to our bodily, animal existence, by contrast with the 'higher functions' that relate to our 'rational' mental lives. The early suffragists of the mid-19th century took a servant class for granted and were primarily concerned with equalizing access to education for what Virginia Woolf was still calling 'the daughters of educated men' when she wrote *A Room of One's Own* and *Three Guineas*, her two proto-feminist manifestos, at the end of the 1930s (Woolf 1935, 1938). Woolf did not regard herself as a 'feminist' and was largely unconcerned about women's political rights as distinct from their access to education, the professions and the life of the imagination; nor did she ponder overmuch on the aspiration to education of lower-class women.

Indeed, much of the drive for women's education and entry to professions in the 19th century addressed the 'problem' of the 'demographic surplus of women' caused by higher death rates among males than females. It was unmarried or 'unmarriageable' women who constituted the 'surplus' – that is, surplus to the marriage market – in each age cohort.

This was mainly seen as a 'problem' for women in the middle classes, Woolf's 'daughters of educated men', who had to remain subject to the governance of either fathers or brothers if they did not marry. Nothing stopped women in the lower classes from working either in the factories and workshops or as the essential foot soldiers of residential domestic service, taking care of the middle- and upper-class families' material and emotional needs. But middle-class 'surplus women', like Florence Nightingale or Eleanor Rathbone, had to confine themselves to voluntary philanthropic activity, somehow get into men's professions or transform lowly 'voluntary' activities like nursing the sick into new professions for women. Rathbone, middle-class daughter of a social reformer, was an active and prominent suffragist and a local Liverpool councillor in the first decade of the 20th century, and in 1929 she broke into national politics becoming independent MP for the Combined English Universities, being re-elected in 1935. Her campaigning, particularly during the Depression, was informed by her awareness of class difference and the needs of the working poor.

What became women's jobs in the paid economy always carried the burden that traditionally they had been done by lower-class women and so were regarded as of lower value and skill than the professions that had traditionally been a male monopoly. They also suffered the devaluation associated with work involving manual effort and/or having direct concern with the body rather than what was thought of as mental or brain work. Even in what became high-status male professions in the course of the 19th century, such as medicine, branches like surgery then carried the status penalty of connotations of manual effort or manual dexterity; still today hospital doctors sometimes jokingly refer to orthopaedic specialists as 'butchers' or urologists as 'plumbers'. And engineering has still not entirely sloughed off the manual/practical connotations that in England (as distinct from Scotland or Germany) have been associated with its non-gentlemanly and practical origins and its Dissenting and provincial provenance.

In the main occupations in which women predominate – such as secretarial and office work and now the routine administrative roles in organizations, nursing, schoolteaching, particularly teaching younger children, nursery work, residential care and other community care work, health ancillary work and social work – both status and income levels suffer from this being 'women's' work. Even efforts to regularize training and raise the value of formal qualifications have had an uphill struggle. Class divisions and gender distinctions dog all attempts to raise such work to the level recognized in economic scales as 'skilled'. This became precisely the concern of much feminist research and campaigning, but none of it has ever effectively shifted the disbenefit attaching to what has been and still remains associated with the traditional female caring role.

The value of caring has also been affected by other social and cultural shifts, which I shall merely indicate here and explore more fully in subsequent chapters. The rapid loss of influence of the churches after the 1960s, more especially the collapse of the traditional socialization of the young into Christian values if not into churchgoing, meant that the sense that caring for others was a particular Christian duty got dislodged. Although many values that had been cultivated through the churches have a shadow life in the increasingly secular world, they have largely become detached from any specific religious anchor and have to sink or swim in a competitive secular cultural market. The ever-increasing value placed on autonomy and the fulfilment of the individual self was given an enormous boost by the effects of the counterculture, first in youth culture and artistic circles, then more broadly and powerfully by the economic models of the free market and the preferences of the individual consumer in the neoliberal economic era. Markets and bohemia in unholy collusion gave selfish self-concern a sharp profile and a good press. Along with increased geographical and social mobility and the differentiation of the occupation structure, old class solidarities and traditional community structures have been placed under pressure and in many places seriously eroded. The Brexit split in the country demonstrates this with unmistakable clarity: the new mobile middle classes in the metropolitan areas voted Remain, while the ageing working-class and predominantly White populations 'left behind' in all the 'red wall' constituencies – which had lost their manufacturing base and faced stressed civic facilities, poor employment prospects and eroding community structures (like the place where I grew up) – voted Leave.

Individualism was exaggerated by the increasing hedonism of the consumer market and of culture. This played a part in weakening the authority of institutions – for example, in politics and education, in cultural judgements of 'taste' and in family obligations. Duty and continuity became dubious values that trammelled the freedom lauded as everyone's right. Although there are undoubted plus sides to these cultural shifts, notably a more inclusive and less censorious view, one consequence of focusing so heavily on 'self' has been to render increasingly invisible the value and necessity of interdependence and caring for others, whether in private life or in the economy, until, that is, COVID-19 briefly shook us all awake.

In the rest of this book, I take a selection of these changes and examine them in more detail. I have been surprised that what I discuss comes back so persistently to issues of secularization. Initially, my intention was to get secularization in Britain out of the way quickly in order to focus on the issue of care. In part, I was afraid of being deflected by a subject, secularization, that had been my husband's lifelong intellectual preoccupation and not unimportant in my own. I should have realized that if you pull at one thread in the social fabric, you will find it is connected to more other threads than you perhaps bargained for. I started from the place where I myself began in my own life, the Christian commandment to care for our neighbours 'as' ourselves; and so the die was cast. The underlying justification of care for others becomes a problem when secularization alters the fabric of culture and erodes the sacred. For which others should 'we' care? Who should do the caring? And at what, or whose, cost? Is caring a dubious and doomed part of the 'ascribed female role'? What part did the sexual and gender revolution play in the story of secularization and in the history of care? These questions address only part of the tangled network of interconnected developments that have altered the cultural fabric. Add in changes in demography, technology, the nature of work, the structure of politics, identity and modern capitalism and you find not a neat linear analysis of cultural change but a complex pattern of entangled causal relations.

In the end, the issues that stand out are: first, why caring remains so persistently a female concern despite half a century of feminist criticism; and, second, why such essential and humanly demanding work as care is still not defined as 'skilled' by economic measures and political values and is so inadequately rewarded. Innovations in artificial intelligence (AI) over the next few years are expected to replace or reduce the numbers in many of the occupations currently defined as highly skilled and paid accordingly. These changes will intensify the concentration of income and wealth more tightly in an ever smaller top echelon while reducing the number of middle- and working-class jobs in the economy. This is why there is so much current speculation among worried economists about how a universal basic income might compensate for these market forces – always provided that the same market forces do not crash the system altogether. The application of AI in the care sector is much less likely to eliminate jobs, which, like most others in the service sector, are predominantly 'person facing' and not susceptible to perpetual 'increases in productivity' as currently conceived, which is why so many of them, especially in social care, are organized on 'flexible' lines with low pay and little security or employment protection. A continually expanding need for care among an ageing population for whom medical science can ever more successfully prolong life will only swell care demands. Far from solving the 'care crisis', these developments can only intensify it as well as bring a further instalment of increased inequality in the most economically advanced economies.

The largest issue of all is how to rectify the injustice baked into the system and culture of care under the current political and economic order. The analysis of the current 'crisis of care' has been the subject of a number of powerful recent official investigations and academic and journalistic books and articles. We are not ignorant about the nature of the crisis. There is even wide agreement among professional observers about what needs to be done about it. It is overwhelmingly a matter of political will. This book will not attempt to duplicate these analyses of our acknowledged crisis but aims to do something different. It is a discussion of the underlying cultural discourses and popular assumptions that have shaped the contemporary crisis of care in Britain and the political and economic culture that defines any real solutions as 'too costly' according to values that are never very explicitly defined or defended. While potential technical and organizational solutions have become clear, the necessary shift of cultural values and motivations strong enough to energize the political process and appeal to electorates, and perhaps more importantly to political party managers and social and economic elites, have not. There is no social movement today to motivate necessary reforms to give priority to better care for the weakest and most helpless in our rich, greedy societies that has anything like the potency and urgency of the campaign against climate change. What we face is a moral and ethical deficiency in political and social life that might motivate the reforms that many people already understand are necessary. I hope the following sketch of the changes in the culture of care that have happened over my long life may point to where some of the blockages lie.

2

Secularization and the Second Great Commandment

Who is my neighbour?

In the local parish church, every Sunday morning throughout my girlhood, I listened to the rector begin the Communion service by reciting either the Ten Commandments or Jesus' summary from the Gospels, the two great commandments: love God with all your being and love 'your neighbour' as you love yourself. Before the bread and wine were offered, we were told that we must be 'in love and charity' with our neighbours. I often thought how much easier it would be to keep the Ten Commandments than to love my neighbour 'as myself'. The parable of the good Samaritan had told me that everyone in the world was my neighbour, and loving all of them that way seemed nearly impossible. It was certainly a tall order for an 11-year-old in 1948, when I began to attend 'grown-up church' as well as Sunday school. Wartime censorship and self-censorship had lifted and some of the war's terrible details had appeared on the radio news and in newspapers – the unimaginable brutality of the Holocaust and, almost worse, the fact that 'we' had dropped two atom bombs on Japanese cities. The second great commandment had implications that were beyond my grasp. Closer to home than my dimly guessed dilemmas of Christian doctrine in relation to war and foreign policy, I agonized in an entirely personal way over my own moral responsibility whenever I encountered casual racist or anti-Semitic remarks, as I often did, especially in the queue at the Co-op grocery shop. 'Dirty little Arab' was the everyday description of a grubby small boy; toddlers crying for their mothers were jokingly terrorized with 'Get away! She's run off with a Black man!'; and at that time in the North West, gentiles colloquially used 'jew' as a verb, meaning 'to cheat' (Boyd 2017, p 132; Jacobson 2022).[1] It was part of women's banter as they counted their change – 'I thought you'd jewed me there!' Should I say something or would that be 'forward', uselessly cheeking my elders and my, literal, neighbours? Both speaking and silence left me tormented.

The morally hyperbolic demand of the second great commandment is a reason why so many people have regarded Christianity as unrealistic and why, in practice, it is regularly trimmed to accommodate normal social necessities. The political historian Peter Hennessy reflects on the history of the phrase 'a duty of care', which after 1948 was applied to the new responsibilities of the state for the welfare of its citizens. The term had originated in a legal judgement in the House of Lords in the 1930s, in a case for negligence brought by a woman against the company that had allowed a decomposed snail to be left in the bottom of a bottle of ginger beer, which had made her ill. The former Lord Justice of Appeal Sir Richard Aikens QC explained to Hennessy:

> The rule that you are to love your neighbour becomes in law, you must not injure your neighbour; and the lawyer's question, Who is my neighbour? receives a restricted reply. You must take reasonable care to avoid acts or omissions which you can reasonably foresee would be likely to injure your neighbour. (Quoted in Hennessy 2022, p xviii)

Sir Richard Aikens uses a phrase from the Gospel accounts of the parable of the good Samaritan, or from the Book of Common Prayer, as the obvious source for a legal term and a judicial decision. Yet despite pragmatic adaptations of this kind to make the principle practicable, the impossible Christian ideal inscribed in the Gospels and the second great commandment is never cancelled or quite forgotten; as my late husband, David Martin, put it, it remains 'on the books' however much it is debased in practice and however few people are still familiar with 'the books'.

The problem

In this and the following chapter, I consider how the second great commandment has fared as Britain has secularized over my lifetime and what that means for a common culture of care. As a child, I learned through the family about the importance of caring for others, especially through my mother's seemingly inexhaustible care for her own and other people's children. But it was given a powerful Christian rationale by religious education in school, Sunday school and church. That Christian formation was still common in the 1940s and 1950s, although today it only touches a tiny and shrinking minority. The institutional church has declined, and the decline may have speeded up when churches were closed during the COVID-19 pandemic. Church attendance and membership of all the churches' ancillary organizations have shrunk drastically; the Christian socialization of younger generations has virtually collapsed, leaving all but a very small remnant of the youngest generations with only the vaguest notions of what Christian faith and worship entail; even the few hymns still roared as crowd chants at football and rugby matches have slipped their religious moorings and been drowned out by 'Nessun dorma' or 'Sweet Caroline'. It seems Christianity has lost the larger part of the cultural and political potency it once had in British society. The Christian meaning of care for others has, at best, been obscured.

Secularization

The experience of secularization and its impact on the value of caring for others is my first focus as I enquire how, and how far, caring for others – including the crucial issues of *which* others and *who* should do the caring – still exists as a shared cultural value. But first I need to clear away misleading common assumptions about secularization. Secularization is not an automatic and inevitable consequence of 'modernity' as some theorists have maintained, although that is no longer the majority scholarly view (Bruce 2011). The habit of belief and churchgoing, along with denominational identities, did not fade away on a predetermined path of evolutionary progress. Secularization is as much a project of human intention and historical contingency as it is the structural effect of abstract processes beloved of sociologists, such as the differentiation of social roles and institutional spheres. All kinds of historically and culturally specific contributory factors have been suggested, including Alec Ryrie's intriguing contention that unbelief grew because early modern Protestant perfectionism made it too emotionally stressful for people to believe 'with all their hearts and minds and strength' (Ryrie 2019). I shall not adjudicate among causes of secularization here but only note the dubious presuppositions of some secularization accounts or rhetorical claims.

The philosopher Charles Taylor notes how humans reach for narrative to make sense of our world even when we think we are appealing to reason or 'science'. He criticizes what he calls 'subtraction stories', on which most secularization theories rely (Taylor 2007). The story is told as if human consciousness in a pristine state (itself a purely hypothetical notion) would have had a blank where historically religion has been printed on it. In a subtraction story, secularization happens when an 'artificial' or 'arbitrary' construct, religion, is swept away and leaves a clear screen or blank slate for modern secular rationality to fill. But human consciousness is never the empty slate or blank computer screen that the metaphor implies, nor is pure rationality its 'natural' state. From birth onwards, the consciousness of every person is shaped by the underlying realities that societies conjure to make sense of the world – sense that is emotional, relational and social as well as 'rational' or 'scientific'. There is no warrant for assuming a secular outlook is more authentic or less arbitrary than a religious one. All societies construct a 'social imaginary' in which they interpret their world through language, ideas, narratives, myths, images and practices that leave a deposit that comes to be taken for granted (Taylor 2003). Abstract reasoning, empirical observation and memories of historical events may feed into it, but so also do all the imaginative arts – poetry, dance, music, ritual, drama, stories, games, sport and humour. Secularization is the replacement of one social imaginary that intimately weaves 'religion' into its pattern by another that replaces it with 'secularity'. Both are inevitably *ideological* since they rest on value premises. Once in place, these value premises become so invisible from customary use that they are unrecognized for what they are; they become 'self-evident' as the original justification becomes hidden or forgotten, so people believe all sorts of things they would be hard pushed to explain.

During five centuries and more of dominance in Western Christendom, Christianity built up a moral framework that was the context from which 'modern' values emerged, including the idea of the secular itself. Charles Taylor explains this as the way the Christian 'sources' of modern moral 'frames', or perspectives, have become 'occluded' – that is, hidden in plain sight – because they have become so 'normal' that they are unquestioned, even in a Western secular age that prides itself on questioning everything (Taylor 1989). Secular society has an inner, and for the most part unacknowledged, Christian skeleton.

Care for others, or more accurately for selected others, may well be part of our evolutionary heritage, since it is a common feature of primates, although among primates care tends to be confined to the immediate group. Our animal heritage has sometimes been interpreted as the evolutionary emergence of exchange relations that involve calculation – 'do as you would be done by' or placation of the powerful – rather than either a strict 'survival of the fittest' or a generalized instinct for altruism (Klein 2014; Hare and Woods 2020; Raihani 2021). Some commentators, in a genealogy that runs through Machiavelli and Nietzsche, believe moral constraints on individual self-interest are a group-induced delusion and care for others is idiocy unless it benefits oneself (Paley 2021). Others, in a tradition of Enlightenment optimism, offer a selectively rosy picture of natural human goodness (Bregman 2020). Yet, however much care for others may, or may not, be part of our instinctual nature, it is never the disinterested duty of care for all others that the second great commandment demands; that kind of virtuoso ethic was a moral innovation of the philosophies and religions of the Axial Age. In the cultural history of the West, a duty to care for others is clearly rooted in the religious deposit of Christianity as are other moral principles that are now claimed as 'secular' or Enlightenment virtues but historically were extrapolated from theological doctrines: the equal value of all humans and the belief in universal 'human rights' sprang from the doctrine of humans 'made in the image of God'.

Charles Taylor calls the modern, secular dispensation of consciousness and language 'the immanent frame' and regards it as the 'default' perspective of modern Western cultures (Taylor 2007). The immanent frame assumes the primacy of the here and now and gives no priority or cosmic significance to the 'transcendent', to ideas about a good that reaches beyond immediate human 'flourishing'. It provides the medium through which a secular social imaginary is generated and normalized in the modern West and is even the title of a website of the US' Social Science Research Council devoted to 'secularism, religion and the public sphere'.

Historical episodes of secularization pose questions about: how far they are driven by ideological agencies and ideas; what the context of structural or contingent historical changes may be; and how these changes reshape the social imaginary. These questions arise in the episodes of secularization in Britain since the end of the Second World War that I outline in this chapter. I select these contingent episodes rather than others because they impinge directly on the value of caring for others, the categories of people who have or do not have calls on our care, and the social and cultural context in which the value of care is embedded.

Secularization in Britain: from then to now

The secular spaces that already existed in my childhood multiplied after the war. My younger siblings, like many others of their baby boomer generation, gravitated to them and increasingly avoided religious spaces as boring or constricting. But for most adults in the working-class culture in which we grew up, life was still organized around religious markers of time and space, the Christian rituals marking birth, marriage and death and the events of communal life that followed the church's liturgical sequence: Advent leading up to the Christmas festivities that ended with the Sunday school pantomime; the indulgence of Pancake Tuesday before Ash Wednesday began the Lent fast; Good Friday, when we all climbed the highest local hill; Easter with Easter eggs; Pentecost, when all the local churches marched through the town In the 'Whit walks' and Sunday school children wore the 'new clothes' that every family somehow contrived to buy for that symbolic beginning of summer (Burns 2013)[2]; harvest festival, which had significance even for urban people at a time during the war and the extended period of austerity after it when fresh fruit and vegetables were only available locally and in season, and milk often still came in churns from nearby farms; and the Methodist Sunday school anniversaries, which sometimes borrowed the best singers from the other churches for their packed performances of Mendelssohn's *Elijah*, Stainer's *Crucifixion* or Handel's *Messiah*.

Secular times and spaces were interspersed with these: the wakes weeks in summer when all the mills closed for the yearly holiday, and the spring and autumn weeks when the fairground came to town or bus and train excursions to the Blackpool illuminations were organized, as well as the escapes from the world of work provided by dance halls, cinemas, theatres, pubs (male) and teashops (female), soon to be joined by the coffee bars of the 1950s. Yet most public and family celebratory moments were still part of the weave of the Christian year. Its ritual markers measured out family life and its calendar acted as a mnemonic for shared memories. Photographs were still rare and treasured records, often taken at one of these festival times; and reminiscences beginning 'Do you remember ...?' were usually placed in context by association with one or other of these Christian seasons.

That ritual marking of the communal year according to the liturgical calendar is now little more than a distant echo, like the folk Christianity that was threaded through working-class community life, even among people who seldom went to church outside 'hatching, matching and dispatching'. Drawn curtains told you someone had died and was 'laid out' in bed or in their coffin for visitors to pay their respects; people stopped and men took off their hats to a passing hearse; and women talked familiarly to the dead in the cemetery. People observed all kinds of purity and boundary rituals that gave them a sense of control over precarious situations. Women like my mother and aunts were 'churched' after childbirth, thinking of it not as purifying their blood-polluted sexual bodies but, as with 'christening', a religious insurance policy for the baby's safety. Almost everyone performed good luck rituals, carrying 'lucky charms' or mascots, performing tasks in a 'lucky' sequence and always sending out the darkest-haired male in the family with a lump of coal in his pocket to 'let in the New Year' on the stroke of midnight on 31 December, with that 'first footing' coming in through the front, never the back, door. This patchwork of ritual and 'superstition' was treated as continuous with Christianity, although most of it had a folk genealogy and no theological warrant. That included the idiosyncratic selection of what counted as 'work' – the tasks that all my churchgoing aunts 'religiously' avoided on Sundays. And whether or not they attended church or chapel, almost everyone had a denominational identity.

Martin Stringer wrote an illuminating ethnography of this culture (Stringer 1999, 2008). In the 1999 book, he provides a vivid account of the admixture of folk beliefs and Christian worship in three Manchester church congregations, mainly using women's experiences. In the 2008 book, he draws not only on his own research but that of graduate students who studied beliefs and practices of this mixed kind in a number of mainly working-class congregations, again mostly with women, in several areas of Britain but prominently in the industrial North West and Midlands. Stringer sees the 'folk religion', or cluster of 'superstitions', that these studies describe as part of a widely distributed pattern interpenetrating, and probably predating, Christianity in Britain and elsewhere. A repertoire of customary beliefs and practices provides contextual resources to supply reassurance and comfort in situations where they seem to 'fit', with no concern for 'theological' coherence or overall consistency and quite distinct from the discipline of erudite or elite 'systems'.

Secularization is the story of how this common heritage within which the Christian message was passed on, mostly enveloped in a buzz of other cultural 'noise', disappeared between my childhood and my old age. The details of the decline of the churches and of Christianity in British life is well documented elsewhere, but accounts of plummeting religious metrics do not do justice to the unravelling of the intricate cultural weave I experienced as the undergirding of everyday life. Current heated debates about the rise of identity politics and the loss of community cohesion suggest that some potent residue of nostalgia for what has been lost in this unravelling may still be at work in ways seldom explicitly acknowledged.

I have two particular questions about the accepted account of British secularization.[3] The first is to do with the extent to which ideological agencies have explicitly given it a helping hand (an issue surprisingly seldom addressed by secularization theory). The second concerns how completely the Christian deposit of values disappeared – specifically, whether the second great commandment, or a pragmatically reduced version of it, has migrated into a cluster of secular values and/or remained distinctively Christian.

Individualism and collective identities

Most secularization commentators agree that one of the drivers of change is the postwar growth of individualism – a value with a long back history in Christian culture (Seligman 2000). Once the collective disciplines of the war years could be relaxed, individualism intensified in the second half of the 20th century. This was the latest stage of what Charles Taylor identifies as the modern self's 'disembedding' from the shared symbolic practices in which it had traditionally been nurtured – family, community, class, gender, ethnicity, nation, region and religion. That 'embedded' character is what I tried to capture in the description of my experience of church and community during my childhood. As the economy opened up after the Second World War, new occupations emerged, social, educational and geographical mobility began a slow then accelerating increase and, tentatively at first, people began to discard the unwritten constraints, obligations and coercive meanings of what had been taken for granted. The freedoms of increased individualism are easy to celebrate and the dubious and, at worst, virulent aspects of collective identities are easy to deplore – the Protestant/Catholic divide in the urban Lancashire of my childhood, which mirrored more violent sectarian conflict elsewhere in Britain, the automatic anti-Semitism and distrust of 'foreigners' and the unthinking racism of citizens of the 'mother country' of the British Empire all illustrate the moral downside of collective identities that render difference threatening. Intersecting cultural movements from the second half of the 20th century selectively teased and seduced people away from earlier collective constraints. Contradictions between the individual and the collective good feed a chronic tension in modern societies. The agents of change include the development of mass secondary and then mass higher education, discourses of feminism and the counterculture, a popularized therapeutic culture focused on the individual self, the growth of mass consumerism and popular entertainment in the postwar era and, more recently, the expansion of communication and virtual connection by ubiquitous digital media. Much of this has either been driven by or opportunistically subsumed into the capitalist profit imperative. All these cultural changes have the potential to set the interests and desires of individuals against the solidarity of older collective identities. Some go further and stimulate new collective identities, often creating 'virtual communities' via electronic media among those marginalized or excluded by traditional structures. All of them can be successfully 'marketized' and/or 'weaponized'.

Challenges to the selective moral blindness of traditional identities have created a new form of identity politics. Sometimes this stimulates reconfigurations of older collective identities, as in the emergence of new forms of ethnocentric or conservative identity. These reconfigurations can be defensive reactions to change, but some spawn a violent fringe, like those male 'incels', who blame all women ('feminists') for their personal failure to find sexual partners, or like aggressive adepts of certain conspiracy theories. Not many of these new 'identities' are intrinsically toxic, but the claims of both old and new collective identities carry cultural and political implications, notably those defined by nationalism, ethnicity, faith, gender, generation and sexuality. Yet today, very few people do *not* experience overlapping layers of identity, which may as easily contradict as reinforce each other. Particularly where the modern 'self' is understood as a continuous, integrated identity, these contradictions can raise questions about what constitutes a self's primary identity, the answer to which will often vary with context. Alternatively, the contradictions may even receive a positive gloss in 'postmodern' conceptions of the 'fluid' or 'fragmented' self.[4] Contradictory personal identities surface routinely in the course of contemporary life – in the family as against in school, with childhood friends as distinct from adult colleagues, between spouses/partners and their respective birth families and so on. A 2021 study of Generation Z in Britain and the US examines the way members of this generation, currently between their late teens and mid-twenties, manage to compartmentalize incompatible identities while building fine-grained individualized ('modular') identities for themselves which can find an online and even offline community of similar others (Katz et al 2021, especially chapter 2). Identities challenge and are challenged by others in an expanding range; whether the rights of biological females (cis women) should be preserved by excluding transwomen from their spaces, as gender-critical feminists have argued, is only one of many such dilemmas. Experiencing disagreements as a threat to the wellbeing or safety of one of the parties is another dilemma that today can lead to the 'cancelling' of controversial speakers, say, in universities. Although most young adults in Generation Z believe in supporting the rights of all self-chosen identities, even those with which they disagree, a morally and politically unambiguous route through rival claims to collective and individual 'rights' and identities is anything but self-evident, and in most cases the difficulty relates to the degree of exclusiveness with which the in-group/out-group boundaries of these potentially warring identities are invested.

This is only an extreme version of the unavoidable tension at the heart of caring, magnified by individualism and the tangles of identity politics, but never absent – the distinction between caring for 'our own', the people in the immediate group, especially the close family, or people we see as 'like us' as against caring for the good of the whole group, or wider society, let alone caring for distant or even hostile Others. One of the familiar temporizing clichés of my childhood was 'charity begins at home', and there were many such sayings that limited care for others within 'sensible', usually meaning affordable, bounds. 'God helps them as helps themselves' was another, familiar long before Margaret Thatcher turned it into a welfare policy in the 1980s. These are part of the folk resources analysed by Martin Stringer. The second great commandment collapses all these distinctions and gives no priority to close kin or to any collective Us over Them, even when They are the 'enemies' whom Christians are, anyway, commanded to love. The parable of the prodigal son does not even expect the wastrel son to become 'deserving' before his father forgives him and throws a celebratory feast to welcome him home. And the person who shows up worst in that parable is the virtuous but resentful stay-at-home son. Charles Taylor, in his Catholic persona, believes that the Gospel vision has been extended in modernity to include equal human rights and to require 'unity-across-difference' (Taylor 1999, p 14). This formula encapsulates the fundamental challenge of the Christian message: it demands the impossible and challenges the normal necessities of power and solidarity. The conundrum is unresolvable outside 'the kingdom of heaven', but on this earth, ways are usually found to fudge absolute moral demands in the interests of social coherence and political viability: neither 'Christian' nor secular states find it politic to behave like the father of the prodigal son. Consider the case of Shamima Begum, the British schoolgirl who had her British citizenship withdrawn after leaving her family and community in East London during her GCSE year to join the radical

ISIS (Islamic State of Iraq and Syria) califate in 2015.[5] Despite her appeals and the defence that she had been groomed online as an idealistic 15-year-old and had voluntarily walked away from the collapsed ISIS caliphate, the British government has refused to accept her back or restore her citizenship as a 23-year-old adult who has been held in a Syrian detention camp for the last five years, because she is still regarded as a potential terrorist risk.

The history of secularization illustrates this kind of dilemma many times – indeed, one definition sometimes employed by my late husband, David Martin, might be expressed as: any socially or politically convenient limitation placed on the second great commandment, especially by the powerful. The following episodes of secularization show the principle of care for 'neighbour' hedged around with contingent and historically specific social and political limits, but sometimes constituting efforts to enlarge those limits in the way Charles Taylor identifies as modern extensions of the Gospel. They also highlight the role of ideological agencies and the ways in which a secular social imaginary has been established as the principle of care for others has emerged in a secular as well as a Christian modality.

Episodes in British secularization and their implications for the value of care for others

Episode 1: Radical theologians of the 1960s as ideological agents

The first episode was an own goal by the churches. It concerns a radical theological movement of the early 1960s that galvanized a discourse of secularization while at the same time yoking it to Christian care for the poor and marginalized. Sam Brewitt-Taylor's research on a movement that has been ignored in most accounts of British secularization shows how a small group of theological radicals took up continental, mainly German, theology that had emerged from the spiritual and political dilemmas facing Christians in Europe between the two world wars (Brewitt-Taylor 2018). Paul Tillich, Rudolph Bultmann and the anti-Nazi Lutheran pastor and martyr Dietrich Bonhoeffer were particularly influential. Brewitt-Taylor thinks the British theological movement they inspired invented of the idea of 'the radical sixties' and gave a sharp impetus to the ideology of secularization (Brewitt-Taylor 2013).

The radicals were concentrated in the clergy of the established church in Britain and in the divinity departments of the universities, but they had counterparts in Non-conformity and in Catholic Europe and America. The movement attracted notice in the late 1950s and early 1960s, and it declared secularization a fact and a desirable goal at least half a decade before churchgoing began any dramatic decline. Radical theology proclaimed a new age in which Christianity would abandon its institutional forms and take its message out into society at large. This would usher in the 'kingdom of God on earth' by breaking down the boundary between church and 'world', sacred and secular, unleashing universal love. Radical theologians and clerics assaulted boundaries, limits and institutions in the name of love some years before it became the slogan of the counterculture. The popular apex of theological radicalism was probably the publication of Bishop John Robinson's bestseller *Honest to God* in 1963. The book stirred controversy by rejecting outdated images of God in favour of an existentialist theology in which God is 'the ground of being', as well as by its sympathetic account of situation ethics. Robinson himself became notorious as one of the expert witnesses for the defence in the 1960 trial of Penguin, publisher of the unexpurgated version of D.H. Lawrence's novel *Lady Chatterley's Lover.* The prosecution was unsuccessful and this led to a revision of the Obscene Publications Act, which will figure again in a later episode.

By the beginning of the 1970s many of the leading radicals had left the church for secular employment, believing 'the world' the proper arena in which to put their ideas into practice. Brewitt-Taylor (2018) takes the Reverend Nicolas Stacey as exemplary. Stacey worked in social outreach and community politics and eventually left the church for professional social work. The influence of theological radicals in the universities continued through their publications and teaching long after the movement had waned among parish clergy. Don Cupitt, for instance, set up the Sea of Faith network in the 1970s to spread his 'non-realist' philosophy of religion from Cambridge, a development that later influenced the 'spirituality' movement.

In the early 1960s, my husband and I wrangled over these ideas with radical Anglican priests and Methodist ministers who wanted to purge the Christian faith of doctrinal and supernatural 'frills' and rid themselves of their 'traditional' congregations. The clergy we knew personally were especially vehement about the 'dead hand' of respectable elderly women and harboured the (quickly deflated) hope of replacing them with the radical young. Despite the biker priests, the coffee bars in the nave, and the youth clubs for 'un-clubbable' teenagers who were already deep into youth culture and its new music, and in spite of serious attempts to reach out to the marginalized, the radical theologians and clergy left many churches as emptied out spaces. These were partly reoccupied over the following decades by a revived evangelical movement. An organizationally weakened Student Christian Movement was elbowed aside in the universities by the evangelical Christian Union. Cathedrals were mainly left to conserve an older choral and liturgical tradition, which was confronted in many parishes by modernizing initiatives and evangelical informality. By the end of the 1960s, the radical theological movement had largely run its course, but it had had a hand in shrinking church attendance, destabilizing Sunday schools and other ancillary organizations by doubting their usefulness, hollowing out the Student Christian Movement and shifting the church's political sympathies to the Left and its moral theology in a liberal direction. The latter provoked a rising tide of confident evangelicals, who often shared the liberals' concern for social responsibility but stiffened conservative standards of personal and sexual morality against liberals like John Robinson. The radical theological episode highlighted the priority of care for those at the bottom, or outside the social hierarchy altogether, as more important than institutional forms, and it sharpened the divide between liberal and conservative Christian views of personal sexual morality.

The theological radicals believed the highest Christian duty was to stand with the poor and socially outcast rather than nurture a closed club of 'insiders' in church. This dramatized the contradiction between the policing role of churches, in patrolling the boundaries of moral and social 'respectability', as against care for the poor and marginalized even, or perhaps especially, when it meant challenging codes of respectability, as Jesus himself repeatedly did. This contradiction exists throughout Christian history and is a recurrent cause of controversy and scandal.

Christian agape *versus respectability*

In his comic epic *Handling Sin*, the North Carolina novelist Michael Malone has theologically serious fun with this contradiction in the spirit of the radical theologians of the 1960s (Malone 1984). His story is set in the racially divided American South in the 1970s and celebrates the radical Christian challenge to respectability. Malone's virtuous hero, a conscientious life insurance broker, is the Baptist son of a jazz-playing White Episcopalian priest who had been expelled from his living for flagrant adultery and attempting to desegregate his church and who then taught in a Black college and trained its marching band. The stuffed shirt, respectable hero conducts a running debate in his head with 'that fool Christ' and his own irresponsible father during the wild goose quest on which his dying father sends him. Malone tells a redemption story in which his rationally moderate everyman is forced out of his cocoon of self-righteousness to embrace a wider human care for others across the boundaries of respectability, race and most of the seven deadly sins and find a new respect for 'the hobo Jesus' as well as love for his wise fool of a father, his own prodigal half-brother and his embarrassing neighbour.

One of innumerable parallels to Malone's moral carnival can be found in a 17th-century song of praise for 'Saint Francis the vagabond', the church motet 'Aqui, aqui, valentones!' (roughly translated as 'Come here, you ruffians') by Juan de Araujo, a Spanish baroque composer working in Peru (see de Araujo 2005). The scandalous inverse relationship between respectability and Christian love, exemplified by Francis of Assisi,[6] was also a feature of liberation theology in Latin America between the 1960s and the 1990s at the time of the juntas. Scandalous contradiction is particularly marked in the 'queer and indecent' theology of Marcella Althaus-Reid, the Argentine radical feminist who saw the face of Christ in the suffering of a tortured street child, a transvestite and a slum prostitute (Cooper 2021). The potential for scandal always lurks in the Christian message championing the 'foolishness' of Christ against the wisdom of the worldly wise.

Episode 2: The collapse of common Christian socialization

There is little mystery about how common Christian socialization in Britain collapsed so completely in the 1960s and 1970s. When the state extended schooling to the children of the labouring classes in the Education Act 1870 and made attendance compulsory in 1880, schools became the main conduit of a nondenominational Christian socialization common to all in more or less mono-religious Britain. This came to an end between the early 1960s and the mid-1970s through legislative and curricular changes inaugurated by educational and political elites.

In the heyday of common religious socialization, churches, chapels, Sunday schools and other ancillary organizations undertook denominational formation, and some families took direct responsibility for the religious shaping of their children. By the early 20th century, that family role was fading. Family prayers and even grace at meals had fallen away, and families increasingly left religious formation to the educational and religious 'experts' in schools, churches and Sunday schools. In 1950, around a third of all under-15s still went to Sunday school, but towards the end of the 1960s, decline gathered pace as it did in the membership of other ancillary church organizations (Thompson 2017). This shrinkage was not unique to religious organizations; secular associations also suffered declining membership and attendance. By 2010, Sunday school attendance had dropped to 5 per cent, and has continued to fall (Thompson 2017). Sunday school teaching depended on volunteer laity with little training, and the church historian Naomi Thompson attributes some of the fall in attendance from the 1960s to their continued emphasis on control at a time when child-centred learning was becoming customary in professional pedagogy (Thompson 2017). Theological radicals questioned the point of Sunday schools. Analysts of British secularization, notably the historian Hugh McLeod, see other social changes at work, such as rising affluence, greater mobility and the appearance of a wider variety of leisure activities as alternatives to the offerings of church associations, especially at the weekend, including football and cricket youth leagues (McLeod 2007, 2022).

Between the early 1960s and the mid-1970s, compulsory religious instruction in schools underwent radical revision that ended the common nondenominational Christian formation. A significant change began in the 1950s with the appearance of more religious minorities among the school population alongside the long-standing Jewish group, particularly in the towns and cities where ethnic minorities had clustered. Although there had long been small enclaves of non-White and non-Christian workers, mainly in docks and shipping, the Aliens Restriction (Amendment) Act 1919 (only repealed in 1971) had controlled immigration during the mass population upheavals after the First World War, with the aim of preserving the supposed homogeneity of Britain. But the Attlee government gave citizens of the British Empire the right to settle in Britain under the new British Nationality Act 1948. Labour shortages in the newly established National Health Service and what had become publicly owned bus and train companies led to government-sponsored recruitment drives, especially in the Caribbean and the Indian subcontinent, whose populations had contributed substantially to the Allied war effort. This introduced significant new ethnic and faith minorities into several British cities, augmented by later waves of immigration in the 1990s from West Africa and after 2005 from the economically poorer countries of Eastern Europe through European Union 'freedom of movement'. In the 2011 Census for England and Wales, ethnic minorities made up around 14 per cent of the population (Office for National Statistics 2022a), and by the 2021–22 school year just over a quarter of schoolchildren in English private schools and just over a third in state schools had an ethnic minority background (Department for Education 2022).

Christian migrants from the Caribbean met both open and implicit racism in the mainstream congregations they first attended and by the 1970s had set up Black-majority churches, many with a Pentecostal character. The presence of ethnic minorities inaugurated decades of controversy over national identity. Arguments over whether faith should have any place in public life also intensified in the 1980s and 1990s, when religion, widely regarded as in terminal decline in Europe, unexpectedly became a hot geopolitical issue following the collapse of the Soviet Union and the revival of national religions that had been suppressed under state communism (mostly forms of Christian Orthodoxy but including Catholicism, Islam, Buddhism and, in the Baltic countries, several varieties of Protestantism) and with worldwide Islamic revival, some of it radical and political, and the growth of indigenous forms of Pentecostal Christianity all over the Global South, many with diaspora congregations in British cities. Britain began to relabel its minorities not as 'ethnic' or 'racial' but as 'faith' communities.

Compulsory religious instruction in state-funded schools was transformed between the early 1960s and mid-1970s from a basic Christian formation to something more like a detached introduction to comparative religion, while specifically Christian religious education became an optional examination subject. In the course of the 1970s, outside the small sector of faith schools, many school assemblies modified their original character (and legal definition) as an act of Christian worship to focus instead on ethical issues, using popular music rather than hymns and Bible stories, or to reflect the festivals and moral teachings of non-Christian faiths. There were also practical constraints. Many of the large new comprehensive schools of the 1970s and 1980s had more students than could gather in one space, so assemblies became less frequent or rotated around, say, different age segments. Change was undoubtedly also a response to the presence of minority faiths and to growing secularity among the school population in some urban areas, as well as to struggles between advocates of multiculturalism and assimilation among educational professionals.

There may well have been some reluctance in Whitehall to sanction new non-Christian voluntary faith schools, because it would have contradicted the inclusive multiculturalism favoured by the political and educational policy makers who wanted to avoid any appearance of faith 'apartheid' in state schools. This was despite the established practice of exempting Jewish pupils from religious instruction in schools and allowing them to attend their own religious classes instead. At all events, by the end of the 1970s, changes in religious education had eroded common Christian formation, opened schools to secular culture as the common denominator and largely moved any teaching of values, including caring for others, out of 'religious' into 'social, personal and health' education. A Radio 4 series on a multicultural comprehensive school, Acton High, in 2021, illustrates the problems as some members of faith communities feared multicultural schools were exposing their children to secular values. In Acton High, these problems resulted in the so-called 'honour killing' of one ethnic minority student and the death of another in gang/drug violence (Ahmed 2021). The effect of the curricular changes may have been (partly) unintended, but it was undoubtedly a secularization resulting from the choices made by an elite cadre in education and government which might have pursued different ways of accommodating non-Christian faiths. Even so, the wider secularization of culture was seeping into schools and affecting the informal milieu of the students and younger teachers, and might well have done so whatever the state of formal religious teaching. Recent research among university students and school pupils shows that the rejection or abandonment of a religious position is largely a response to influences, not just in families but in school and society, including social media, but also to the individual reflections of children and young people themselves (Strhan and Shillitoe 2019). Strhan and Shillitoe further argue that the failure of religious education in schools to connect meaningfully with the experiences of nonreligious children or to discuss nonreligious materials now amounts to a denial of social justice (Strhan and Shillitoe 2022).

Episode 3: Secular humanists as successful ideological actors

The third episode concerns a small group of secular humanists who influenced not only the changes in religious education just outlined but also the liberalization of laws controlling personal and public morality. An opinion survey for *New Society* in 1965 found that almost two-thirds of parents still wanted schools to give children the basic grounding in Christianity they had received themselves (Goldman 1965). Despite this lack of grass-roots demand, secularizing changes were made. Reviewing data on 'the long 1960s', Clive Field comments on the *New Society* article and a small handful of other opinion findings: 'Humanists and secularists were dismayed by the apparent acquiescence of the public in general, and parents in particular, in state-sponsored religious instruction' (Field 2017, p 17). It touched on a contentious issue for an increasingly vocal secularist lobby, which Rob Freathy and Stephen Parker investigated (Freathy and Parker 2013). Their research shows that, just as Clive Field suggests, secularists and humanists, who had gained increased public notice and some popularity in the 1960s, had put pressure on the consultations on the curriculum of religious education between 1963 and 1975. Although they failed to eliminate state-funded religious teaching, a small cadre of committed secularists and humanists lobbied energetically and managed to get a parliamentary debate on the subject. This outraged some conservative Christian groups, yet religious educationalists welcomed the involvement of secularists and humanists in the curriculum consultations. Freathy and Parker show how senior Christian educators went out of their way to construct curricula that would suit teachers and pupils from every shade of religious or secular opinion and to include secular and humanist philosophies as well as non-Christian faiths in religious education syllabuses. For some, this may have been based on realism, or perhaps sympathetic Christian concern for other faiths, or even a prudent move to head off attempts to remove religion altogether from the school curriculum, as humanists wanted. The presence of powerful advocates for secular humanism together with fraternal consideration for non-Christian minority faiths clinched the case for curricular change by the mid-1970s. A lobby of self-styled 'traditional' Christians, led by Baroness Caroline Cox, eventually succeeded in getting the Education Reform Act 1988 to reaffirm the religious traditions in Great Britain as in the main Christian. The Act reiterated the requirement for religious worship in regular assemblies, although that probably made little difference to established practices. The content and conduct of religious education is now determined by local Standing Advisory Councils on Religious Education, which are obliged to take account of the ethnic and faith composition of local schools.[7]

Recent research in America on the success or failure of religious socialization shows that the crucial factor for success is parents and their parenting style (authoritative but not authoritarian, relaxed but not laissez-faire, with consistent conversational engagement with their children on religious matters; Smith and Adamczyk 2021). The American context is different from the British one in constitutionally separating church and state, which means providing no religious education in the main school system and expecting religious families and churches to take direct responsibility for it. It is hard to imagine that between the 1970s and the end of the century many British parents would have engaged proactively in effective religious socialization, whatever the school religious curriculum had been.

Secularist pressure also scored a notable success in influencing policies regulating personal and public sexual morality. The historian Callum Brown's *The Battle for Christian Britain* is an openly partisan account of how a small elite group of committed humanists took on the entrenched influence of the churches in a campaign to liberalize the laws of public decency, public and private sexual behaviour, divorce and abortion in Britain between the 1960s and the 1980s, overturning the privileged role of representatives of the churches (Brown 2019). Brown acknowledges that churches were mainly represented by religious 'conservatives' on influential policy and advisory bodies. The Central Religious Advisory Committee of the BBC and the British Board of Film Censors (which became the British Board of Film Classification) influenced the policies of national and local bodies on the licensing of public performance spaces and rules affecting pubs and clubs. Conservative church people, mostly men, had for many decades operated their own pressure group politics inside the churches as well as in public life, at a time when new theological ideas were already filtering into many religious bodies and bringing more liberal perspectives to sexual and gender issues. This occurred in such seeming redoubts of tradition as the Mothers' Union (Moyse 2009; Jones 2013). By the 1970s, the strict conservative stance of religious and moral 'culture warriors', like Mary Whitehouse and Malcolm Muggeridge, was no longer representative, if it ever had been, of the opinions of the laity or even of non-evangelical clergy and ministers. By the time the reforming Labour Home Secretary Roy Jenkins got liberal changes to the laws on divorce, abortion and homosexuality on to the statute books in the second half of the 1960s, and with his reform of the Obscene Publications Act 1959 liberalizing its operation after the *Lady Chatterley* case, the humanist lobby had seen the end of the monopoly influence of religious conservatives in this area.

Episode 4: Educational distributors of a secular social imaginary

In *The Battle for Christian Britain*, Callum Brown refers to the increasingly secular assumptions in teaching, the BBC and the mass media from the 1960s onwards (Brown 2019). A 2016 Reuters study of journalists in Britain illustrates the point. It revealed journalists as less Christian and more, and more profoundly, disbelieving than the general population. In the 2011 Census, 59.3 per cent of the population identified themselves as Christian and 25.2 per cent as nonreligious (Office for National Statistics 2021), while the overall proportions were reversed for journalists in the Reuters study (Thurman et al 2016, especially pp 10–11). By the 2021 Census, the general population had moved closer to the journalists (Office for National Statistics 2022b). David Goodhart, at least by implication, agrees with Callum Brown about the increasingly secular assumptions of the media and education, particularly in universities (Goodhart 2020). He criticizes the contemporary imbalance between 'head' (conceptual and analytic skills), 'hand' (physical and artisan skills) and 'heart' (emotional intelligence skills) in the jobs market and sees the postwar rise to dominance of occupations requiring a university degree, and the abstract thinking it rewards, as responsible for the decline in the status and dignity of both manual and artisan work and of care occupations, or 'heart work', somehow reflecting the rise of secularity and the decline of religion. He writes: 'The Head world is generally a secular one with little feel for the mysteries of life, which is why so many of us today seek a substitute for it in everything from yoga and meditation to the green movement' (Goodhart 2020, p 279). This may be little more than Goodhart repeating 'what everyone knows', but that, in itself, illustrates the taken-for-granted secularity of the contemporary university and the 'cognitive' jobs for which it prepares students.

A little discussed source of cultural secularization in tertiary education is the often aggressively secular complexion of burgeoning university departments of sociology and other social sciences, as I experienced them at the time. The sociologist of religion Grace Davie makes a similar observation in assessing the research evidence about secularism and secularization in postwar Europe: 'European social science was – and in many ways still is – a profoundly secular enterprise' (Davie 2022, p 272). The 1960s saw a large expansion of higher education and the foundation of a group of new universities. Departments of social science were among the fastest growing up to the mid-1980s, and they figure prominently in the hinterland of the leading humanists cited in Callum Brown's (2019) study, such as Baroness Barbara Wootton and the abortion law reformer and sociologist Madeleine Simms. Departments of social science sent their graduates into the expanding occupational sectors best placed to shape public opinion, especially on issues of care.

Social work is the most obvious case, as its business is the care of many of the most vulnerable. Between the wars, a few colleges and universities offered diplomas, but in the 1960s and 1970s social work became an increasingly professionalized graduate sector. Social work training was usually located either in departments of sociology or in new departments of social policy or social administration and modelled on the pioneer courses developed by

Professor Richard Titmuss at the London School of Economics and Political Science as part of the infrastructure of the postwar welfare state. Social work had originated mainly in religious and philanthropic initiatives and in the 1960s still had a small cadre of committed Christian teachers, mostly older women, who were gradually replaced by younger social scientists. Titmuss himself was religiously agnostic and his department at the London School of Economics and Political Science was popularly known as the 'Department of Applied Virtue'. This was a jokey put-down in which the notion of virtue was used with an edge of secular sarcasm to draw attention to the normative nature of the discipline; its focus on care for the needy was not sufficiently 'objective' or 'detached' to qualify it as a 'real' science.

The founding fathers of the social sciences had all worked within an Enlightenment intellectual framework and an evolutionary model of 'stages' of society in which religion characterized the lower and earlier stages to be superseded by secularization in the highest stage, today or at the latest tomorrow, through inevitable 'progress'. The secular orientation of sociology and other social sciences was taken for granted but justified, if challenged, by this need for 'scientific objectivity'; it was popularly argued by leading sociologists of religion, for example, that all research in the subject must practise 'methodological agnosticism'. It took until the 1990s for the majority of social scientists finally to accept the methodological and philosophical case that all observers have an inescapably 'situated' perspective which inevitably inflects their frameworks and the questions they pursue as well as being liable to influence the responses of the subjects they are observing.[8] The secular temper of sociology went with it into offshoots like medical sociology and criminology and into the aspects that entered the curricula of other academic disciplines from medicine and law to literature. In the 1980s, nursing went through a development very similar to social work, becoming an all-graduate profession with a substantial strand of medical sociology in its training and care as its rationale. David Goodhart, for one, sees the conversion of nursing in the 1980s to an all-graduate profession as an instance in which 'heart' skills – that is, empathetic caring skills – were demoted in favour of 'head' skills, making senior nurses into quasi-doctors or health administrators at the same time as eclipsing the earlier religious rationale of the work (Goodhart 2020, pp 217–23).

Social science graduates took the secular perspective into other expanding professions such as social research, market research, opinion polling, public administration, teaching at all levels, counselling and therapies of many kinds, the law, and the media, including journalism. This was a conduit through which Charles Taylor's 'immanent frame' was normalized and the social imaginary steadily secularized among the expanding numbers of the university educated and the opinion formers in the expanding mass media. At the same time, social science graduates, including many from the baby boomer generation, tended to absorb ideals of social reform, sometimes used ironically, as we saw in relation to social policy and social work, but nevertheless feeding political ideals and many varieties of radicalism enshrining secularized liberal, socialist or Marxist principles of social justice.

Summary

These incidences of secularization as a conscious project – Sam Brewitt-Taylor's account of the secular eschatology of the radical theologians of the early 1960s, accelerating secularization in the churches; the decisions in state education that dismantled common Christian socialization; the success of a small group of secular humanists in overturning the privileged influence of conservative church representatives in religious education and the legal control of public and private morality; the role of the expanding departments of social science as key distributors of a secular perspective, particularly to fast-expanding professions that prominently include modern modes of popular communication as well as the caring sector – together suggest contingent and often contradictory collusion between differently motivated initiatives. They all strengthened the *narrative* or *discourse* of secularization together with the secular social imaginary embodied in it. By a significant paradox, they also gave a stronger emphasis to caring for others, including protection of ethnic/faith minorities, both in the churches and in the public realm, most particularly in the operations of the postwar welfare state. They strengthened anti-racist and egalitarian opinions as an application of the imperative of caring for others, especially among the growing numbers of graduates. This merged with the liberal, critical and Left-leaning secular schools of thought that tended to dominate the curricula of most of the social sciences, with the conspicuous exception of economics and some versions of political science. In these ways, the developing secular social imaginary began to shuffle the moral principle of care for others between the religious and the secular ledger.

3

Care for Others, Secularization and Britain's New Identity Tribes

The secularization of the value of care?

This chapter begins to explore the effects on the value of caring for others when secularization at least partly dislodged it from its historically Christian root and justification to make it a self-evidently 'secular' value. A throw-away remark in Alan Johnson's memoir reflects what has become a common observation: 'as the country has got less Christian in its religious adherence it has become more Christian in its way of life' – that is, more caring and less casually brutal in its attitudes towards minorities of all kinds, whether to do with race, sexuality, disability and so on (Johnson 2018, p 23). Alan Johnson was one of the few genuinely working-class Cabinet ministers in the Tony Blair government after the 1997 landslide victory for Labour. In the later stage of the Blair administration, between 2006 and the Party's defeat in 2010, Johnson served as Education Secretary, Health Secretary and Home Secretary. He was part of the team that boosted the welfare state just before the financial crisis of 2008 put on the brakes, used as the rationale for George Osborne's austerity policy in the following Conservative–Liberal Democrat coalition government. Alan Johnson's verdict on the changes he had observed over his lifetime (he was born in 1950) is the view of a moral optimist who can see an 'occluded' Christianity still at work in society's values and in political action, including the politics of the Labour government of which he was a part – though Alistair Campbell, atheist spin doctor to the Catholic convert Tony Blair, is reported, at the height of the controversy about Blair's part in the invasion of Iraq in 2003, to have advised his boss, 'we don't do God'. Yet, as secularization began to inflect and limit the understanding, and ultimately even the common memory, of the second great commandment, the priority of care for others has progressively been exposed to competition with economic, political and other secular principles based on very different premises.

Secular value or 'occluded' Christian virtue?

In *British Gods,* Steve Bruce, the doyen of 'hard' secularization theory, revisits a group of classic community studies in Britain from the 1950s and 1960s to bring evidence of secularization up to date (Bruce 2014, 2020). Bruce suggests the people still attending churches are probably more committed to Christianity than was the case when more people went to church but were only nominally Christian. In a long-running controversy with Grace Davie, he insists that the residual respect for the clergy still found in many communities, notably so in the aftermath of local and national disasters, illustrates the 'impotence' of today's clergy rather than, as Davie argues, being a sign of 'vicarious religion' – Christians acting as proxies for the nonreligious (Davie 2006). Bruce writes: 'Were the churches still powerful more people would resent them' (Bruce 2020, p 67). He goes further in the same passage, reflecting on cumulative opinion poll data: 'Although organized religion enjoys considerably less prestige than it did in 1900 or 1950 church people are still taken to be honest, decent, caring and non-partisan' (Bruce 2020, p 67).

The vast majority of the British, a majority growing with each successive generation, are not much interested in the Christian faith, have little or no knowledge about it and regard attempts to promote it as at best embarrassing and at worst an assault on individual autonomy. Yet they still see Christians as admirable when they do things for others – run or support food banks and charities, set up fair trade stalls, campaign for refugees, tend to rough sleepers, use their churches as hubs of community support in crises, including the COVID-19 pandemic and the influx of refugees after the 2022 invasion of Ukraine by Putin's Russia. That's just what Christians do, as indeed do other faith communities, and what they are expected to do by their religiously indifferent fellow citizens. However, for Bruce, the value of caring for others is obviously a *secular* matter, just ordinarily decent.

Bruce's insistence, even more than Alan Johnson's opinion, is a textbook illustration of Charles Taylor's (2007) claim about the 'occluded' Christian frame of secular modernity, including in relation to universal 'human rights'. The problem with occluded frames is that the justification for any particular value can be forgotten along with its origin once it becomes self-evident. This can give moral philosophers well as policy makers, lawmakers and social activists, considerable difficulty if they ever have to make consistent sense of what are assumed to be shared 'secular' values. The value of caring for others runs up against limits even in the most coherent modern systems of philosophical and ethical thought, such as Alasdair MacIntyre's virtue ethics or John Rawls' theory of justice. Limits assert themselves in the case of Christian arguments too. In his 2022 Reith Lecture on 'Freedom of worship', Rowan Williams, retired Anglican Archbishop of Canterbury, maintains that debates about the value of religious freedom are fundamentally concerned with 'the kind of beings human beings are in a world just as this one is' (Williams 2022). Religion, he believes, is uniquely placed to challenge those convictions we uncritically inherit from the consensus of previous generations because 'moral conviction is … the argumentative grit of the worshipping community'. Moreover, worshipping communities are able to bring first-hand experience to policy issues 'that work on abstractions'. In a clear Christian application of the second great commandment, Williams urges Christian communities to press on 'issues of unequal power' to insist on human dignity and protect the most vulnerable.

The Christian principles of William Temple were part of what underpinned and motivated the Beveridge welfare developments in Britain after the Second World War, yet however much Christians may share Williams', or Temple's, general conviction about the Christian priority of care for others, disagreements inevitably arise over how it should apply in the real-life circumstances that confront individuals and groups with problematic cases. This occurs, conspicuously, over whether some kinds of maldevelopment of the foetus are so severe as to justify abortion – that is, for the sake of the foetus itself, whether a woman has the right to choose what happens to her body and her life, and whether her wellbeing and even survival are more or less important than those of the foetus. Many decades of controversy within and outside organized religion have been spent on such problems with no overall consensus. In the public commitment to care, the problem is at its clearest in relation to the severely disabled, where no version of the secular utilitarian calculus can justify care for them. What principle of utility or overall happiness could justify the life-long, full-time care of a child who can never become a self-sustaining adult – care given, say, by a parent who perhaps also has a demanding job and/or other children to care for? Whose life is more 'valuable' there? Valuable in whose eyes? And what more 'productive' use could be made of the resources consumed in such care by the welfare services and/or the parents of such children?

The historian Margaret Spufford wrote about confronting these problems as a Christian in the 1960s when she gave birth to a daughter with a life-limiting condition who needed constant care. Together with her husband, she chose to give first priority to caring for her daughter and fighting for resources to prolong and enrich her child's life and the lives of others like her, while herself suffering chronic and crippling ill health (Spufford 1989). Frances Young, a contemporary British Methodist theologian, wrote about her now-adult son with severe learning disabilities. When Arthur was born, her urgent sense that he ought to be valued and cared for *because of* his total helplessness and despite his evident 'uselessness' could not be validated by any secular philosophy, and certainly not by a liberal philosophy in which mature, rational exchange was the central assumption of the social contract (Young 2014). Unlike Margaret Spufford's daughter, whose cognitive development was normal, Arthur is unable to offer reciprocity in the usual sense or to give rational assent to his treatment or arrangements for his care. His mother found that no secular philosophy could value his acute disability as anything other than waste, much as the ancient Spartans would have done. For Young, only the Christian theology of creation could make sense of 'a world gone wrong'. The image of the crucified Jesus enabled her to see in her son's broken body and mind an image of Christ's brokenness. His disability was the key to Arthur's integration as part of the whole body of the human community rather than the insurmountable obstacle to it. She only found peace when she stopped agonizing about how to reconcile the goodness of God with the reality of evil and random disability and simply got on with being 'alongside' her son's suffering rather than yearning, or even praying, for its healing or miraculous reversal, as some of her Christian friends urged. She began to see Jesus' expiation of human sin in his suffering not as a kind of 'legal transaction' but about

> the kind of love that stays with our pain, with the anguish of hearts before the inexplicable mysteries of life, with the suffering of innocents, with the absence of resolution in the face of tragedy. That 'staying with' rather than 'putting right' is a perception deepened by living with irremovable disability. (Young 2014, p 121)

States do not run on such rationales when deciding who deserves their care; they reach for the utilitarian and prudential.

The problem of justifying care for people who cannot care for themselves and can never, or can no longer, 'pay back' society suggests that the hidden skeleton of Christian values may still play a part in triggering the supposed 'gut' or 'instinctive' reactions of some people, perhaps specifically of mothers, to value and care for the helpless and damaged members of family and society even when they are not convinced Christians. The folk saying 'only a mother could love him/her!' encapsulates a once common view of just how capacious maternal love was thought to be. Penny Wincer is another professional woman who chose to care for a severely autistic son who needs full-time attention. She gives no indication in her account of having any religious motivation for accepting the intermittently distressing and always exhausting life that choice entailed (Wincer 2020). The severity of her son's needs had unfolded slowly so that she had already spent a decade of loving and caring for him before the full extent of the difficulty became clear. Maybe she never felt the need to consider the abstract question of what underlying religious or secular value justified his care; it could simply be taken for granted.

All three of these women took primary responsibility as mothers, but they all received valuable support from husbands in the work of care, even though

Penny Wincer and her husband divorced and lived separately. (Couples with disabled children are proportionately more likely to divorce or separate than couples without such children, although there is wide disagreement about the exact statistics.) Even when mothers manage to continue to work, as all three of these professional women did, they need considerable help even beyond what partners contribute. If the 'responsible parent', who is usually the mother, has no partner to share the care and no paid employment, she is at the mercy of the adequacy or otherwise of public provision.

The problem of how to justify costly care funded by the state or charities or, always, by the formally invisible labour of unpaid family carers who are overwhelmingly women, will recur as my argument unfolds. An intrinsic justification for the individual and social costs of care is not often explicitly considered. Yet it underlies the relation of caring and gender and the persistence of the implicit duty of care still resting on women, and widely internalized by them, particularly as mothers; and it affects welfare policies and practices where budgets have to be politically and administratively decided and defended. In the care sector of the British welfare state, the claims of those needing continuous personal care – notably, those with severe learning difficulties and those suffering advanced dementia – run up against the chronically inadequate provision that demonstrates the low level of priority that, in practice, such people are afforded.

I make these observations to draw attention to the hidden consequences for public policy as well as for political and social culture at large when policy rests on an implicit, supposedly 'secular' notion of the value of care that leaves the 'duty of care' nakedly exposed to economic, financial, political and sectional pressures. These pressures operate according to competing and not always coherently justified criteria that today have largely superseded the unconditional moral protection of the most vulnerable, which has for long been provided, at least in principle, by the impossible but compelling moral Christian universalism of the second great commandment. The secularization of values has hidden consequences.

Care for others as the mark of a Christian?

Religion shows itself in ways of living and dealing with 'all the ills that flesh is heir to' – such as death, suffering, injustice – but in dealing with all the joys and satisfactions too. This kind of perspective may be as significant as measuring religion by assent to creeds and articulate beliefs. A 'lived religion' framework of this kind is the underlying premise of Grace Davie's conception of vicarious religion. The chapter she wrote with Nancy Ammerman for the International Panel on Social Progress in 2019 expresses it succinctly: '[lived] religion has as much to do with navigating social life as it does with the supernatural' (Ammerman and Davie 2019, p 44). It is important to keep this in mind in considering the hazards and ambiguities of secularization. After all, there are many varieties of secular culture, most of them coloured by the religions against and through which they are defined.

Although he regards care for others as, now, a self-evidently secular value, Steve Bruce is right about it also being publicly recognized as the special mark of Christians in Britain. In the short run, the cultural changes of the 1960s and 1970s turned the Anglican Church into what was often described at the time as the only effective opposition to the Thatcher government in the 1980s, standing up for the marginalized when the Labour Party was preoccupied by an internal struggle between the centre and the hard Left. The hard Left had considerable clout in some still-powerful trade unions and in the local politics of large cities, including parts of London and Liverpool, at the point when modernizing and free trade policies weakened trade unions and accelerated the closure of mines and the failure of much of traditional manufacturing and heavy industry in the old industrial areas. The established church still retained a considerable, if reduced, reservoir of moral authority at this time, which it exercised through its bishops in the House of Lords (Hatcher 2023), through the monarchy (the monarch is still Head of the Church) and through clergy and laity in local communities, including what Ammerman and Davie call the 'street level' ecumenism of all denominations working together with other faiths (Ammerman and Davie 2019, p 34). Significantly, this has often meant the Church of England providing an umbrella for non-Christian minorities on whose behalf the established church made public declarations and representations on issues of human rights and immigration to the governing administration in local government as well as in the Lords. (The coronation of Charles III in 2023 was the first time that leaders of non-Christian faiths took a direct part.) In the 1980s, the Church exercised its moral authority and still significant social clout on behalf of ethnic and faith minorities, the poor in the inner cities and those who found that the industries on which their communities had depended were run down or closed across what was fast becoming the 'rust belt' of Britain. The report of the Archbishop of Canterbury's Commission on Urban Priority Areas, *Faith in the City*, was politically controversial but widely influential (see Davie 2017, pp 53–9).

One chapter in this story is told in *David Sheppard: Batting for the Poor*, the biography of the celebrated England and Sussex batsman and crusading evangelical Bishop of Liverpool in the 1980s (Bradstock 2019). 'Race' is at the heart of this episode. As a cricketer, David Sheppard took a stand against apartheid by refusing to play against the all-White South African team on their 1960 tour and protesting against the Marylebone Cricket Club's proposed tour to South Africa in 1968–69. As Bishop of Liverpool from 1975, he became closely associated with his Roman Catholic counterpart, Archbishop Derek Warlock. The two worked indefatigably for the improvement of housing and social conditions in the inner cities in the 1970s and 1980s, and frequently challenged the policies of the Conservative government. Archbishop Warlock applied the principles of Catholic social teaching in this collaboration, notably the priority of 'putting the human person first' before economic or political interests. Their work influenced Jenny Sinclair, Sheppard's daughter, who converted to Roman Catholicism after bringing up her family. In 2011, she founded a charity, Together for the Common Good, to 'combat individualism and foster social trust in and between communities' by encouraging everyone to take personal responsibility for the common good and for the renewal of civic ecology.[1]

Social outreach and conservative moral rules: British evangelicals

As the example of David Sheppard, a leading evangelical in the Church of England, shows, this focus on care for others, with its political implications, was not confined to the lingering effect of the theological radicals or the theologically liberal wing of the Church. It also marked the growing evangelical wing, even though the evangelical approach to family, gender and sexual morality placed it in the 'conservative' camp. The Roman Catholic Church showed the same combination of conservatism on sexual and family morality and progressive political stance on social justice, after Vatican II in particular – its British constituency was dominated, in any case, by people of Irish working-class origins. From the 1960s, the clergy and ministers of all the Christian churches, especially their national leaders, along with the British and the World Council of Churches, became increasingly engaged by social outreach, issues of social justice, global and national poverty and inequality, racism, immigration and, eventually, problems such as climate change and population movements that affect the whole planet. The same shift was found in the faster-shrinking Nonconformist denominations. Evangelical churches in Britain are found in Nonconformity and in the Church of England and as independent congregations. They are strikingly unlike the politically Right-wing phalanx of evangelicals in the Republican states of the US. British evangelicals roughly align with Left-of-centre causes, even many that remain 'conservative' on personal and sexual morality. In the Church of England, the laity has remained somewhat more politically conservative than the clergy and on average more liberal on issues of personal and sexual morality, but overall, since 1945, the Church has gradually but decisively lost its 19th-century reputation of being 'the Tory Party at prayer'.

A study published in 2020 by Ruth Perrin about Christian millennials, those in the generation born during the early 1980s and the mid-1990s, corroborates the picture of the collapse of Christian socialization but also of the continued moral and spiritual importance of care for others (Perrin 2020). It also illustrates the evangelical flavour of such churches as do still attract younger generations. Only 3 per cent of millennials identify as Christian and the proportion is even lower in generations after that (Katz et al 2021). The research on Generation Z finds that most have had no serious exposure to religious socialization and construct their identities according to the personal characteristics that are most salient to them, notably sexuality, gender, race and ethnicity (Katz et al 2021, pp 67–8). Churches that still attract a substantial proportion of young adults tend to be independent congregations with an evangelical or even Pentecostal character, upbeat, informal worship styles and close, supportive, family-friendly congregations. Perrin's small sample from England's urban North East is virtually indistinguishable from the nonreligious majority in most ways other than in their faith. Even those with a denominational upbringing have retained little or no knowledge of Christian doctrine or history. They do not defer to authority and they expect to be involved in organizational decisions. They value 'authenticity' and personal fulfilment, which for Christian millennials includes finding a 'romantic' relationship leading to marriage and a stable family. They expect faith to supply immediate solutions to problems at work and in relationships. Most distinctively, they frame their lives around altruism and social justice, confronting poverty, marginality and global problems such as environmental degradation and climate change. For a small number, often men, this can entail considerable financial and career sacrifices. By contrast, young mothers often suffer isolation and difficulty caring for young children unless they have local family support. This split between intimate care in the family, which falls to women, and care for distant others in the name of social justice, often taken up by men, illustrates a familiar gender division which will be important as my argument develops. Research on Christian university students also shows their tendency to search for employment and social milieux compatible with their Christian social and ethical outlook and indicates that they can find it hard to reconcile this with the ambition assumed in their educational context. This is particularly true in the precarious labour markets many of them currently face. Choosing the ethical option is often a luxury afforded more easily by those with support from affluent backgrounds or by women seeking work in the care system, charities or not-for-profit companies (Guest and Aune 2017).

Summary of religion and secularization in 2020s Britain

Before looking at changing social divisions as they relate to the value of care for others, let me summarize the pattern of religion and secularization in 21st-century Britain. The 2021 Census for England and Wales found for the first time a minority claiming to be Christian, 46.2 per cent down from 59.3 per cent in 2011; 37.2 per cent chose 'no religion', up from 25.2 per cent in 2011 (with a particular increase in Wales and in the North West);

and 6.5 per cent stated Muslim identity, up from 4.9 per cent in 2011 (Office for National Statistics 2022b). The 'no religion' category is internally rather incoherent, covering atheists, agnostics and 'spiritual'. London remains the most diverse multifaith and multicultural city but there are now places in the Midlands, notably Leicester and Birmingham, where there is a roughly equal proportion of different ethnic/faith communities and no dominant Christian group. The 2021 Census for England and Wales found 10.1 per cent of households containing members from two different ethnic identities (Office for National Statistics 2022a), a fact which may contribute to explaining how government education statistics report that over a third of state school pupils in England (37 per cent in 2024; Department for Education 2024) have an ethnic minority background despite these minorities accounting for 14 per cent of the population (Office for National Statistics 2022a).

A particular issue has been highlighted in relation to those choosing 'no religion' in 2011. Social scientists have pointed out that in this year the Census question on religion asked respondents to choose from a list of faiths, with 'no religion' at the bottom but with 'Muslim' second in the list, immediately after 'Christian' (Day and Lee 2014). This may have triggered an 'ethnocentric' response from people who felt the need to assert their inherited 'native' or national Christian status as a form of 'White' ethnic identity to mark their difference from 'immigrants', particularly Muslims. This accords with my early experience of nominal religious identities in the working-class communities of the urban North West. It also fits Steve Bruce's interpretation. He notes that most opinion surveys find practising Christians markedly more favourable to serious religious people of any faith, as distinct from 'those people who adopt the Christian tag as justification for their xenophobia' (Bruce 2020, p 175). A version of 'xenophobia' appears again as White ethnocentricity in emerging new 'identity tribes' in Britain.

In the wake of the 2021 Census, a survey of 5,000 nones by the Theos think-tank filled out the picture of people who currently regard themselves as having no religion – referred to as the 'Nones' (White 2022). The Theos sample found the under-50s were proportionately more likely than older people to choose 'no religion'. It also found some incoherence within the category. Only 51 per cent of nones did not believe in God, and 42 per cent thought there was some form of the supernatural. Hannah White divides the nones into three distinct clusters with various degrees of knowledge and opinion about religion, God and spirituality. 'Campaigning Nones' made up 34 per cent of the sample, and the majority (68 per cent) were men. They were mainly atheist and actively hostile to religion. Much like the New Atheists of the early 2000s, they tended to see science as the only reliable form of knowledge and, like Richard Dawkins, condemned religion for having a malevolent influence. 'Tolerant Nones' made up 35 per cent of the sample. This group had the highest level of education, was relatively evenly composed of men and women and had a tolerant rather than a hostile view of religion, based on a 'live and let live' principle. 'Spiritual Nones' made up 32 per cent of the sample, and the majority (61 per cent) were women. This group believed that 'humans are at heart spiritual beings' and tended to be hospitable to New Age ideas, such as belief in ghosts, angels, the healing power of crystals, reincarnation and the power of prayer.

A contradictory patchwork of belief and unbelief has a long history in the British population, going back to the time when a majority was affiliated in some sense to a church or chapel, so this sort of tangle is hardly novel: Martin Stringer's argument discussed in the previous chapter is relevant here. Research on British religion from the 1950s onward has found that beliefs in life after death, or in reincarnation, or in the power of prayer seldom show a consistent relation to each other, to belief in God, to churchgoing or to Christian identity (Martin 1967, pp 74–6; Abercrombie et al 1970; Stringer 1999, 2008). It is not surprising, then, to see in the Theos sample 20 per cent of nones believing in life after death but only 11 per cent in the existence of heaven, 16 per cent in reincarnation and 17 per cent in the power of prayer, or even 6 per cent still saying grace at mealtimes.

An earlier Theos report by Nick Spencer, *Doing Good: A Future for Faith in the Public Square*, has apposite observations on these inconsistencies (Spencer 2016). Five years before the 2021 Census, Spencer found an extraordinary kaleidoscope of plural belief and unbelief. Although the nones were not yet so numerous and Christian identity still covered over half the sample, the trends were already clear. What Spencer believes they show is the 'default' position passing from traditional 'Christian' identity to 'no religion', a projection corroborated by the 2021 Census figures. Spencer is clear how much of a muddle the none identity is, just as 'Christian' identity has long been a melange. Spencer cites a 2008 Theos survey in which only 12 per cent of adults showed a good knowledge of the Christmas story, and comments: 'The common Christian culture into which virtually every English, Scottish, Welsh and Northern Irish person has been born for the last millennium is passing, to be replaced by a confusing plural patchwork *haunted by strong Christian associations*' (Spencer 2016, p 24, emphasis added).

This Christian haunting is partly reflected in the inconsistent mixture of beliefs that has a long back history in folk Christianity. It is also evidenced by the increased prominence of Christian social action. In *Doing Good*, Spencer offers an alternative narrative to the familiar jeremiads about imminent Christian disappearance. He shows recent decades as a period of growth in the social action initiatives of the churches. In 2016 faith-based charities were 50,000 out of the total of 180,000 charities in Britain and the number had grown markedly over the previous decade. 'There may be fewer Christians but they are doing more' (Spencer 2016, p 44). Faith-based charities accounted for 23 per cent of the £16 billion charity income in

Britain in 2016. That sum dipped during the economic difficulties that accompanied and followed the pandemic but the dip has affected secular at least as much as faith-based charities. Social action by faith-based charities, for Spencer, represents 'embodied neighbourliness', 'a way of finding God and worshipping him in others' (Spencer 2016, pp 54, 13). A comment in *The Church Times* on a television documentary about the Black comedian, actor and dramatist Sir Lenny Henry suggests the hidden religious influence of such 'embodied neighbourliness'; the reviewer notes Henry's own tribute to the influence and support of his parents in his career, but the programme makes no reference to the 14 years when his mother sent the young Lenny to Sunday school, which the reviewer sees as the unremarked backdrop to Henry's 'multi-million pound charity efforts' and the star's insistence on a worldwide concept of 'neighbour' (Gray 2023, p 30).[2]

Another aspect of the continuing importance of the Christian churches is perhaps so obvious as to be easily overlooked. This is the value of 'the plant' and the often secular community uses to which it is put. A report from the National Churches Trust estimates that the annual contribution church buildings make to the wellbeing of communities, in terms of social and economic value, is some £55 billion, calculated according to HM Treasury Green Book guidance (National Churches Trust 2020). Church buildings have been key places for rebuilding communities after the COVID-19 pandemic and act as meeting places for all kinds of social activities, religious and secular, for charities and organizations, and as the locus of food banks and warm rooms in the cost of living crisis; they are 'the social glue that keeps our communities together' (National Churches Trust 2020, p 5).[3] It is a moot point whether this counts as Christian or secular on the ledger for the extent of secularization.

New identity tribes: the evidence of the Brexit vote

The 2016 UK Referendum on Membership of the European Union revealed changes in the political salience of cultural identity among the British population. A hostile or ethnocentric response to ethnic minorities is a crucial part of this change, affecting churches as well as the nonreligious population. Some immediate interpretations of the voting figures in the religious press rushed to judgement on its significance for the churches. People who self-identified as Church of England predominantly voted Leave (Clements 2017), although a prominent group of bishops had campaigned for Remain. One journalist argued that the laity of the Church of England had 'tipped' the balance in the vote (Taylor 2018). Left-leaning priest-journalist, Giles Fraser, claimed the Church had 'lost its flock' over the referendum, also pointing out that the Leave-voting laity tended to be more liberal on issues of sexual and public morality than Remain-voting (evangelical) leaders such as Archbishop Justin Welby (Fraser 2018). Cooler, more systematic analysis of the religious correlates of voting in the referendum shows something more nuanced. Ekaterina Kolpinskaya and Stuart Fox, in a study of religion and Euroscepticism, found that it was nominal Christians, particularly non-practising Anglicans (self-identified as Church of England), who were disproportionately likely to vote Leave, while Roman Catholics, whether practising or not, were disproportionately likely to vote Remain (Kolpinskaya and Fox 2021). Yet, overall, attending any church and having active religious beliefs and devotional habits was positively associated with tolerance and concern for migrants and refugees – that is, characteristics associated with Remain voters. Opposition to Europe, defence of British sovereignty and conservative cultural and nationalist values were associated with, but not exclusive to, purely nominal, never-attending, self-defined Christians, above all those describing themselves as Church of England (Kolpinskaya and Fox 2021); this is consonant with Steve Bruce's observation about White 'xenophobia' presenting as nominal Christian identity (Bruce 2020).[4] Kolpinskaya and Fox found characteristics with the potential for religious effects on the referendum vote – religious self-identification and/or belief and/or religious behaviour – in as much as 60 per cent of the British population (Kolpinskaya and Fox 2021). Around 20 per cent of the overall population with any kind of religious identity had characteristics associated with voting Leave, and 25 per cent with voting Remain. The kind of religious involvement made a difference. The more active and committed the faith, the more caring for others had political implications that involved positive attitudes to migrants and foreigners.

The voting in the 2016 referendum provides evidence of the transformed social and political geography of what Maria Sobolewska and Robert Ford call Britain's new identity 'tribes' (Sobolewska and Ford 2020). These tribes coalesced gradually as the pattern of social divisions gradually transformed after 1945 away from the class-based ones that defined party politics after the introduction of universal male suffrage in the late 19th century. Manufacturing and heavy industry had been in decline for nearly three decades before the precipitous collapse under the Thatcher economic restructuring of the 1980s, but the expansion of white-collar, professional and managerial employment after the Second World War eventually transformed Britain from an economy with a large base of manual workers to one in which the much-expanded finance sector, knowledge economy and services form the central core. The idea of class acquired fuzzy boundaries in this process, which substantially affected the emergence of the new tribes.

The expansion of higher education supplied the 'credentialized' manpower and, increasingly, woman-power of the postindustrial economy. In the first few generations after 1945, university expansion acted as a motor of upward social mobility that was easily absorbed by the expansion of the white-collar and professional sector without any substantial balancing downward mobility. Upward social mobility had slowed almost to a stop by the 1980s and may even have gone into reverse by the 21st century, particularly after the financial crash of 2008. Yet the expansion of higher education, with a short pause in the 1970s, has continued inexorably and has played a crucial part in the new pattern of social divisions. When I went to university in the mid-1950s, only 4–6 per cent of my age cohort entered any kind of higher education and women made up less than a quarter of them, fewer if teacher training colleges are excluded. The percentage of school leavers going to universities rose to about 10 per cent in the 1960s. Today more than a third of school-leavers go on to higher education – 35.8 percent in 2023, down from 38 percent in 2021 – and women now constitute a small majority – 57 percent in 2023 (Bolton 2024; HESA 2024).

Peter Mandler describes this expanded higher education as democratized (Mandler 2020). David Kynaston believes that higher education has now become a recognized necessity of the decent life rather than a tool of personal mobility and societal economic advance as it was believed to be in the 1960s and 1970s (Kynaston 2021). The expansion of higher education has clearly been part of the emergence of women as an identity group, partly propelled by grievances about gender inequalities in opportunities and wealth. Some contemporary commentators see the whole education sector as ossified, a failed meritocracy with an obsolete paradigm which has been further damaged by the effects of the pandemic on educational effectiveness and examination assessment. In the view of Matthew d'Ancona, for instance, social mobility and expanded higher education today neither guarantee equal opportunities for children in disadvantaged communities and ethnic minorities, nor provide a sufficiently flexible, critical or technically and digitally literate workforce and citizenry at a time of transformative technological innovation that includes AI, which is already beginning to transform the world of work in a radical fashion (d'Ancona 2021). Adrian Wooldridge too believes that, despite persistent claims to the contrary, there has been no real meritocracy in Britain except for a short period in the reconstruction years after 1945. He describes education today as a misleading melange of plutocracy and meritocracy in which the rich can buy the education that ensures the success of their children, which is nevertheless represented as earned merit (Wooldridge 2021). Selina Todd also sees social mobility largely as a myth which, especially since the financial crisis of 2008 and the years of austerity that followed, belies the widespread reality of stress and anxiety about navigating the uncertainties of the life course to reach some secure achievement (Todd 2020). In 2023, the British government recognized that the disruption of education during the pandemic widened the inequalities of achievement between the top and the bottom of the socioeconomic hierarchy documented in several studies in the preceding years (Jeffreys 2022; see also Institute for Fiscal Studies 2021). Despite all of this, there is some evidence that substantial amounts of short-range mobility have become normal as a large majority of children enter jobs at least one level higher or lower on the socioeconomic scale than those of their parents. Significantly, this level of mobility has been mostly downward in recent decades. Long-range mobility from the bottom to the top of the scale is rare and declining as the number of top jobs has ceased to expand and may even have contracted in recent years (Bukodi and Goldthorpe 2018).

David Goodhart's view of the current overvaluation of cognitive-analytic skills in the occupation structure belongs in this catalogue of critiques of an overexpanded higher education system (Goodhart 2020). He believes that the emphases and values of contemporary higher education have created an undue dominance of cognitive-analytic skills over other types of skill, and that education in the 21st century has not been an effective agent of social mobility. It fails a substantial minority of graduates, who find themselves consigned to routine white-collar and service sector work below the level of their formal educational credentials. In addition to these cumulative critiques, there is widespread disquiet at the way British universities have been 'marketized' – that is, turned into quasi-commercial, or, sometimes, fully commercial markets in knowledge – in ways that squeeze out disinterested scholarship and the values of public service in favour of 'impact' and short-term economic relevance (Collini 2012, 2018; Brown and Carasso 2013; Jones 2019).

The academic consensus seems to be that the postwar education system in Britain has not been any guarantee of social justice in educational opportunity and has not made effective inroads into social and economic inequalities. Nevertheless, the vast expansion of higher education has undoubtedly been important in the emergence of new identity divisions in Britain and in the reduced salience of the language of social class in political rhetoric and popular consciousness. Opinion poll and voting data show graduates of higher education as typically liberal in their attitudes to migration and ethnic minorities. We have already noted that the 'Tolerant Nones' in the Theos sample who were indifferent but tolerant towards religion, were also those most likely to have higher education, which again links liberal social attitudes to higher education.

The presence of ethnic minorities in Britain is a very significant factor in the emergence of new identity tribes. Sobolewska and Ford plausibly divide Britain after Brexit into two main blocs of 'identity conservative' and 'identity liberal', the latter divided between 'principled' and 'necessity' liberals (Sobolewska and Ford 2020). The identity conservative group is made up of an elite of graduates plus a larger group, predominantly people who left school at the minimum leaving age. The principled liberal group is made up of mainly university graduates, which now include growing numbers from ethnic minorities. The necessity liberal group mainly consists of members of ethnic minorities for whom liberal principles protect their community interests. Sobolewska and Ford argue that opinion polls and electoral behaviour reveal migration as the litmus test dividing identities. Attitudes towards ethnic minorities mark the boundary between conservative and liberal. A strong working-class presence in the conservative group is indicated by the majority having left school at the earliest possible point – that is, in the main, the non-mobile White working class, who remain in the communities in which they grew up and who outnumber a smaller privileged traditional elite.

David Goodhart's critique of the dominance of a new knowledge class dependent on the expansion of higher education emphasizes the way that the residential nature of the majority of higher education institutions in Britain has acted as the first stage in the flight of graduates out of their home communities to take jobs and make their eventual homes in large metropolitan economic hubs (Goodhart 2020). In an earlier book, *The Road to Somewhere*, Goodhart divides the British population between this geographically and often educationally mobile, largely graduate group, which he calls the 'Anywheres', from the stay-at-home, non-mobile and largely non-graduate 'Somewheres' (Goodhart 2017). The Somewheres cling to their roots and their marginalized and intensely local identities in provincial towns and rural areas, and they form the bedrock of populist movements in a backlash against the dominance of the Anywheres and their cosmopolitan 'achieved' identities and liberal values. This division cuts across the traditional Left–Right or class division and is the key to the Brexit vote. It was dramatized by the shift of traditionally Labour constituencies in the North into seats won by Boris Johnson's Conservatives in 2019 – the transformation of the 'red wall' into a new 'blue wall' (which then turned back again in the Labour landslide in the election of 2024).

In continental Europe it is far less common for students to go to universities that require them to leave their home areas.[5] Goodhart expresses considerable empathy for left-behind communities and their desire to preserve dignity and respect for their work and the provincial way of life that they believe has been devalued by the rise to prominence of the cognitive elite of Anywheres. Goodhart's morally finessed analysis is very unlike Steve Bruce's dismissive use of 'xenophobia' to describe the same phenomenon, or even the 'ethnocentric' label used by Sobolewska and Ford, which is obviously meant as merely descriptive but nevertheless carries an unacknowledged negative charge in an academic report published from the intellectual heart of Anywhere. Goodhart, however, is less concerned to award moral brownie points than to make sense of what are novel and still inadequately understood social conflicts and political rivalries.

Class versus cultural criteria in the new divides

The importance of class in shifting and complicated interaction with ethnic and religious dimensions is an important part of the picture but difficult to pin down precisely. Kenan Malik probes this in his dissection of race and racism in Britain (Malik 2020). For example, he provides a thoughtful historical reminder that not everyone in the British working classes has counted as 'White' ever since a vocabulary of skin colour became current in the colonial age. In the early 19th century, industrial labourers were sometimes described as 'negroes' by analogy with American (African) slaves, while Irish (Catholic) navvies were caricatured as bestially subhuman or racially Other. Only at the late Victorian and Edwardian height of the British Empire did local British status categories begin to include the working classes unequivocally in the 'White' category as evidently 'superior' to the Empire's subject peoples. These identity labels have a long history and a fiercely contested legacy.

Malik provides detailed analysis of the ambiguous and contradictory interweave of colonialism, race and class in *Not So Black and White: A History of Race from White Supremacy to Identity Politics* (Malik 2023). He traces the historical moves by which 'race' effectively came to mask class interests in labour relations and politics more widely. He recalls how as a young man in Britain, he came to 'unshackle' his own politics from his ethnic 'identity' when he was involved in Indian migrant worker protest movements in the 1970s and 1980s. This showed him how intricately 'race' issues were bound up with wider struggles against inequality and oppression, including those based on class. Malik argues that the exploitations of colonialism fundamentally clashed with the liberal principles on which post-Enlightenment polities in the West claimed to be founded. Slavery contradicted freedom and equality, so racist categories and arguments were invented to justify 'White supremacy'. This occurred not just in slave-holding territories but in societies like Britain that saw themselves as liberal and democratic but had economies and systems of inequality that depended materially on the Black slavery kept at arm's-length in their distant Imperial possessions. Malik teases out the historic and contemporary difficulties of disentangling the toxic distinctions that history has left, and sees them reappearing in new guises in contemporary identity politics. The heart of the problem, as he sees it, lies in the way many sections of the British working class from the 19th century onwards came to see the problem of inequality in cultural terms that represented 'the working classes' as White and as having interests separate from working people of other races and colours (one might add other religions). This division weakened the labour movement and for long has blinded it to its own and British society's prevalent racism. By the 21st century, the rhetorical emphasis on cultural, in particular racial, divisions rather than class divisions had reshaped electoral behaviour in ways that made it half-plausible to proclaim the end of class politics. It was in seeing the marginalization of the working class and its politics as a *cultural* rather than an *economic* issue that the mischief was done. Malik summarizes: 'The more the working class was marginalized, the less class was employed as a lens through which to understand social problems. As class declined as an explanatory tool, culture increasingly became … the medium through which social issues were refracted' (Malik 2023, p 274). This led to what Malik sees as disastrous identity politics. For racial minorities, identity-based solidarity erases distinctions within communities, and for the White working class, it makes them more hostile towards immigrants and minorities. Malik locates the crucial mistake as singling out one characteristic to define the whole identity, even though identity is always more various, layered and contradictory than any one aspect can encompass. Rooting identity and difference in history and culture rather than race and biology is no solution either.

Identity politics makes it difficult to recognize shared characteristics that are more important than ethnic or cultural ones for the purpose of challenging the structures of oppression and inequality – namely, shared ideals and values. Instead of politics that champion one particular criterion of solidarity, Malik recommends 'radical universalism', which might enable people to reattach the economic to the political in challenging inequalities of all kinds. This defence of radical universalism rather than narrow identity solidarities can apply across the whole spectrum of identity politics even though Malik's specific case foregrounds race and class inequalities.

There is clear compatibility if not direct continuity between the Christian moral principle of the second great commandment and the secular liberal support of minorities of all sorts and the promotion of equal human rights of the kind championed by Kenan Malik and Rowan Williams alike, although it is also important to remember the demurs of David Goodhart about the dominance of a (liberal) cognitive elite at the expense of 'hand' and 'heart' workers. What is intriguing is exactly how an expansive understanding of 'neighbour' came to be accepted as the axiomatic secular-liberal position. Research on the influences, secular and religious, on students is relevant here (Guest 2017). It was also a strand in what Kenan Malik experienced as the amelioration of racism in Britain away from the 'vicious and visceral' way it was 'woven into the fabric of society' during his boyhood in the North West in the 1970s (Malik 2023, pp 1–3), as was evident in Alan Johnson's experience in London a decade earlier and in my own childhood and adolescence earlier still. The role of higher education appears to be active in this change, including the diffused cultural impact of the predominantly liberal or radical assumptions in the social sciences and humanities, since, according to Sobolewska and Ford, higher education marks the difference between a conservative identity and a more inclusive or cosmopolitan liberal identity (Sobolewska and Ford 2020). My own values were formed long before I went to university, and Alan Johnson, a notably tolerant Labour politician, never attended university, so it is important not to claim too much for higher education in this respect.

The tone of the mass media also plays a part. The graduate elite among the conservative identity group is not uniformly opposed to migration; indeed, as Sobolewska and Ford report, a virulent response to migration like that of Enoch Powell in the late 1960s and 1970s is rare even among the privileged layer of the conservative elite (Sobolewska and Ford 2020). Yet Powell was dramatically effective in making opposition to immigration rather than shared class interest the key to conservative identity among the White working class, a group prominent among the losers in economic change. The Enoch Powell moment seems to have galvanized that crucial shift from class to cultural difference that Malik identifies and deplores. That includes religious difference. Hence the purely nominal Christian identity among many working-class conservatives that seems to substitute 'Christian' for 'White'. The Israel–Hamas war in Gaza from 2023, in which the death rate of Gazans has been very high, has fuelled protests against the military actions of the government and military of Israel in many Western countries, including Britain. Muslims of all classes have been prominent, but they are alongside other protesters, including Jewish ones. In the 2024 general election, they cost the Labour Party votes and a few seats in urban constituencies in the North and the Midlands with large Muslim populations which had been Labour strongholds. Substantial numbers of electors among ethnic minorities and their radical sympathizers switched their votes from the Labour Party to protest candidates because of Labour's reluctance to support calls for a ceasefire, which occurred as the Party was only just emerging from a drive to eliminate anti-Semitism from within its ranks. Global politics clearly plays a part in the growing instability of party political allegiances and is likely to continue to do so.

The overall size of the conservative identity group and the proportion of graduates in the group declines in each new generation according to Sobolewska and Ford (Sobolewska and Ford 2020). The voting record in the 2016 referendum shows Remain voting, higher education and acceptance of migrants increasing in each younger age cohort. Yet the conservative identity among the old and new working class gave Boris Johnson the victory for Leave and the Conservative Party a landslide majority in the 2019 election, just before the pandemic. This support melted away in 2024, but party allegiances are no longer dependable, as the Israel–Hamas war has clearly demonstrated. Cultural identity seems largely to have trumped class interest and rendered party politics unstable. The extreme caution of the Labour government after the 2024 election in promising to address the crisis in health and social care by reforms but without substantial new expenditure or tax rises is, at least partly, a recognition of this new volatility among the electorate. So far, it does not bode well for care services.

The duty of care in Britain's new identity tribes

Among the identity tribes, different boundaries are drawn around who deserves care, how and by whom. As social analysts begin to rethink the implications of contemporary identity politics, this raises new problems for the economy of care. The bulk of 'identity conservatives' (with important exceptions among its graduate elite, who have never uniformly opposed immigration) implicitly draw the boundary around the people they see as like themselves – that is, mainly White ethnic British, sometimes including White people from the Commonwealth, but leaving ethnic and faith minorities and 'foreigners' of most kinds outside. It is not that this group repudiates the principle of care for others, just that the people who primarily warrant care at the expense of British taxpayers tend to lie inside the boundary of the group, and their welfare is understood as threatened by competitors from outside it. This is an issue for the small anti-immigrant 'populist' parties that have appeared recently, partly fuelled by a realization that Brexit did not solve the 'problem' of the existence of ethnic and faith minorities in the British population (Guest 2022, especially chapter 3). For the 'identity liberal' groups, the duty of care stretches beyond their tribe and often entails care for the whole planet. The value of caring is important to all the new identity tribes in principle, even though in reality everyone draws pragmatic limits – even principled liberals may exclude the illiberal – and, moreover, accepting a value does not guarantee that you will always act on it.

A study of Gen Z, in their teens to mid-twenties in 2020 when the research, by Katz and colleagues, was carried out in Britain and the US, adds fresh contradictions and conundrums to the picture. For this generation, who never knew a pre-digital world, *individual* identity is their major preoccupation or life project, at this stage of their lives at least (Katz et al 2021). Members of Gen Z use digital media to 'discover' who they are and, crucially, who they choose to be, by linking up with digital 'communities' with which they share characteristics they see as important. The aspects of identity that matter most to them are gender and sex, both of which for Gen Z tend to be multiple and fluid, and ethnicity, which is often more ambiguous than has been traditionally assumed, particularly given the many gradations of skin colour and facial features. Members of Gen Z are acutely attuned to differences of wealth and privilege but seldom express them in the idiom of class. From their participation in multiple online communities, they select salient elements from which they build individualized 'modular' identities, taking for granted none of the ascribed characteristics inherited from their background.

Their values are more extreme versions of those held by the millennials studied by Ruth Perrin (Perrin 2020); they focus on authenticity, self-determination and care for themselves and others. Gen Z is conspicuously shorter on religious faith than even the millennials, but does not dismiss it outright, especially in the guise of 'spirituality' (Katz et al 2021). Substantial numbers think they may choose to explore faith later in their lives. They accept and are prepared to defend the freedom of all 'authentic' identities, even the ones they do not agree with, in the name of everyone's right to choose their own values and identity. Although this looks highly individualistic, Katz et al insist that it is always embedded in the chosen community and in a common preference for collaborative rather than isolated individual work practices. Much of this is digitally accessed rather than, as Gen Z expresses it, 'IRL' (in real life). The principle of care for everyone's right to freedom, including freedom of expression, is cited as part of their defence of 'cancel culture', presumably on the grounds that no one has the right to violate anyone else's 'freedom' by confronting them with ideas they find offensive. Yet their championing of a universal right to freedom of expression can sometimes also mean they tolerate 'hate speech' as something that experienced digital users have learned to live with and as a necessary corollary of universal freedom. Coherence and consistency, apparently, are not primary considerations any more than meeting and debating face to face with those who question or challenge their chosen views.

Members of Gen Z prefer to be continually in touch with others, whether digitally or by physical presence; for instance, they still value time with parents and family and often prefer face-to-face relationships (Moran 2023) – witness, the outcry against the suspension of face-to-face teaching among indignant university students whose courses occurred largely, or exclusively, online during the pandemic; and they avoid both silence and purely individualized choices, activities and work practices. How these values will ultimately fare has yet to be seen, particularly if, as is likely, they encounter inimical forms of power and coercion in later adult life. Whatever their views may be at this moment, they will be subject to either the requirements of the profit motive, for those who choose to be start-up entrepreneurs, or employers, for those who take up employment as adults. At this point, however, the preference of Gen Z for nonhierarchical relations and group rather than individual work practices seems to fit neatly with post-COVID-19 technology-based modes of work and organization. In a review of the study, Joe Moran, a professor of English whose students are part of Gen Z, argues that some of the traits exhibited by them are manifestations of long-term trends, including 'greater emotional candour and empathic connection', while others may simply be life cycle effects (Moran 2023). The lengthened stage of adolescence and delayed adulthood of this cohort may be less a sign of long-term cultural change than the economic consequence of the current difficulty of finding secure employment that pays well enough to make buying or renting a home or founding a family feasible. Economics, and the vagaries as well as the continuities of capitalism, can seldom be discounted when we think we see autonomous cultural change. At all events, the importance of some version of care for others appears to be a, perhaps not wholly consistent, core assumption of Gen Z at this point in their lives, although the practical and political implications of their constellation of values have yet to work themselves out. The problem of caring for those who cannot care for themselves is not yet so urgently present for them as it is for their elders.

COVID-19 and the value of caring: is the NHS Britain's real religion?

The COVID-19 pandemic brought an outpouring of support and appreciation for front-line carers, a substantial proportion of whom came from ethnic minorities, according to the press reports of the time. The value of care for others appears to have floated free from its Christian anchor (and from parallel anchors in non-Christian faiths) and, *pace* Steve Bruce, has indeed become a widely accepted value throughout the British population. It might even qualify as the primary 'British value'. How, and how far, its implications differ from the unlimited obligation of the second great commandment will be a recurrent question for the future of care in this country.

The acclamation of carers during the first wave of the pandemic focused on the NHS, and it was not the first such demonstration. At the opening ceremony of the London Olympics in 2012, Danny Boyle, an English film and television director, staged a spectacular opening ceremony that prominently featured a dance routine by NHS workers, which has been broadcast frequently on various media in subsequent years. The ceremony was widely praised as displaying the best of Britain to the world. Frank Cottrell-Boyce, the scriptwriter for the ceremony, commented that in the preparation, 'Danny had built some kind of Utopia, a society run on goodwill' (Cottrell-Boyce 2012). Cottrell-Boyce, a writer from a working-class Roman Catholic background in Liverpool who became Children's Laureate in 2024, made a direct link to Christianity: 'yes, this is a fallen world but you can find grace and beauty in its darkest corners' (Cottrell-Boyce 2012). In the same year, in the introduction to a collection of research essays on religion in Britain, sociologist of religion Linda Woodhead, who a decade later was one of the team responsible for the Gen Z research by Katz et al, suggested it would not be absurd to regard the NHS as the real religion of this increasingly secularized country (Woodhead 2012, pp 21–2). Woodhead was not the first to entertain the idea; most media commentators trace it back to 1992 when Nigel Lawson used it sarcastically, sneering at the pretensions of the medical profession as its 'priesthood' (Toynbee 2018; Lawson 2023). Woodhead repeated her own positive gloss on the notion in the religious press after the pandemic began in 2020, commenting that in face of 'a biblical plague' the British turned not to the churches but the NHS 'to reinforce collective identity … deal with evil and suffering' and 'reaffirm hope' (Woodhead 2020). The idea seems to have become a truism by the time of the COVID-19 pandemic. In early December 2020, Ian Hislop, satirist and editor of *Private Eye*, used it as a quip on the BBC satirical programme *Have I Got News for You* and Jonny Dymond repeated it on *World at One* on Radio 4 on 5 March 2021, reporting the threat of strike action by nurses in response to the Chancellor's recommendation of a meagre 1 per cent pay rise (later increased to 3 per cent but not enough to stave off strikes in response to the precipitous rise in inflation in 2022–23, producing a government-imposed higher settlement, though not high enough to compensate for inflation).

If it is a truism, it is one with a dark underbelly that showed itself as the long lockdown of the first pandemic year disturbed a small minority who vented their frustration and anger on carers. Some of them probably believed conspiracy rumours about COVID-19 being a hoax, some were 'anti-vaxers' and some objected to the curtailing of liberty, but many expressed hostility to NHS carers because of their perceived parade of 'saintliness'. The press widely reported in the autumn and winter of 2020–21 that a small number of hospital workers, including doctors, healthcare assistants and porters, were attacked or subjected to abuse on social media, and toward the time of Captain Sir Tom Moore's death from COVID-19 at the age of 100, his family met a torrent of bile on social media about the celebrity he had gained raising £33 million for NHS charities. (The £33 million did indeed go to its intended charities, but a controversy about the charity set up in his name and run by his daughter and son-in-law filled the media for a year or more and resulted in a ten-year ban on the couple becoming charity trustees.) The shoppers who stripped the shelves of supermarkets to stockpile their own supplies at the start of the pandemic had starred in their own 'me first' or 'us first' story. Caring for others 'as' for oneself is clearly not always accepted as an unalloyed virtue, especially when times get hard. An unknown proportion of the population gives the principle no more than lip service, though even that suggests a need to endorse a virtue valued by most. Substantial numbers have been inspired to volunteer their services in response to the many ways that the pandemic has revealed or intensified hardship, not least some heroic pastors and priests supporting addicts, rough sleepers and the poorest communities (BBC News 2020; Fleming 2023). A similar response has been demonstrated in the willingness of the British population to offer homes to refugee Ukrainians following Russia's invasion of Ukraine in 2022, though many observers have commented on the contrast between this generosity to White Europeans 'like us' and the meagre response to the plight of African, Afghan, Syrian and other refugees fleeing famine, war and civil war beyond the boundaries of Europe.

Of course, the fact that people value and depend on the NHS does not make it a religion. It is a secular bureaucracy with funding, staffing, scope and structure under the control of governments and so subject to the vagaries of political and economic winds. In his history of the institution, Andrew Seaton does not treat the NHS as a religion, but sees it instead as the repository and symbol of what he calls 'welfare nationalism' that sustains the principles of postwar social democracy against the economic advance of neoliberalism (Seaton 2023; see also Hennessy 2022). Yet, even the principle that it should be 'free at the point of need' does not dictate that the NHS should be funded entirely through taxes rather than partly or wholly by some form of insurance system, as many successful and better-resourced European health systems are. The NHS was in crisis almost from the moment it was created, dependent on a partly hostile medical establishment and experiencing a persistent staffing shortage that left it, as it still is, deeply dependent on migrant and ethnic minority doctors, nurses, health assistants, cleaners and cooks from what was the British Empire. After 1948, many of the poorer urban areas would have been without GPs but for the Indian and Pakistani doctors who had been kept out of more desirable and lucrative posts by the pro-White racist practices of the medical establishment (Olusoga 2023).

Even so, the NHS seems to symbolize some quasi-sacred residue of the second great commandment in the British public mind, as illustrated by the frequent references to the NHS as 'our British religion' on all sides of the debate about government welfare spending in the straitened times of 2023. The ritual gestures of the 'clap for carers' in 2021, the rainbow pictures in the windows and the lighting of candles, even the wide public support for striking nurses and junior doctors in 2023 make it a good candidate for Grace Davie's vicarious religion (Gill 2023). But this disguises problems. With the exception of doctors and consultants, who are among the best-paid professionals in Britain, most of the carers receiving these unaccustomed tributes were low-paid and routinely assumed to have little status and minimal skill – junior nurses and ancillary nursing staff, social care workers (the latter not part of the NHS), porters, cleaners, hospital cooks. The caring they do is their paid employment and during the pandemic many of them brushed off thanks with 'We are just doing our job', even though it had often involved unusually stressful effort and long hours in distressing and dangerous conditions. For a brief moment, there seemed to be general consensus that these people are not rewarded by the decent incomes their work, human skill and responsibility warrant. They care for the needy on behalf of us all. But the low status and poor remuneration of the care sector is a historical legacy of caring having been 'women's work', much of it 'manual' labour, which therefore is assumed to need no special skills and for centuries was done without pay or formal training, as indeed much 'informal' care still is. If the very modest pay rise imposed on nurses in 2023 and the relegation of a social care plan to a delayed and financially inadequate place in the government programme are any indication, there is no immediate political prospect of righting this injustice.

Since the height of the pandemic, in light of her participation in the Gen Z research, Linda Woodhead has revised her view about the NHS as *the* secular religion of Britain and now sees the popular reverence for the NHS as only a limited strand in a wider ethical universalism. The title of her 2021 Cadbury Lectures is *Values Are the New Religion* (Woodhead 2021). In the first lecture, Woodhead argues that values have superseded religion in British culture: British Values has even become a compulsory element in the school curriculum, largely taking over the former role of compulsory common Christian socialization. Woodhead believes there is a widespread ambivalence about Christian ethics and argues that much of the population is disillusioned by the institutional churches, Catholic and Protestant alike, which are seen as repressive, preachy and hypocritical. Not all Christian values have been jettisoned along with the institutions, but Woodhead maintains that liberal Christian ideas, including the importance of caring for others, are now subsumed within a secular ethic of universalism. She quotes the figures from the Gen Z study about the relative importance of care for others and care for self: for almost half the sample (48 per cent) the two had equal importance, while 28 per cent gave care for self the first priority as against only 18 per cent who put care for others first (Woodhead 2021). The judgement of the independent individual takes over from that of religious 'authorities'. Woodhead summarizes the change in two pithy soundbites: instead of the old Christian ethic of sacrificial altruism, or 'Give your life!', the British, particularly the youngest generation, now affirm the individualistic this-worldly mantra 'Live your life!' Care has now to be based on mutuality rather than selfless service, and self-fulfilment is everyone's right.

Woodhead's thesis underlines an issue that will be important in the following chapters: the contradiction between the aspects of Christian values that have carried over, selectively, into the contemporary culture of care and those elements of institutional Christianity that are widely condemned for being 'repressive', 'preachy' and 'hypocritical' (Woodhead 2021; Brown and Woodhead 2016). The bulk of what has been rejected relates to official judgements on personal morality, particularly sexuality and sexual relationships, and focuses on the traditional role of the institutional churches as (hypocritical) guardians of moral respectability. This brings into focus a problem that we have glimpsed without yet confronting: the role of sexuality and gender in the secularization process and its consequences for the culture of care. The next chapters will examine this more fully.

4

Caring, Gender and Secularization: The 'Feminization of Piety' and Its Legacy

Contradictions in the principle of care for others

The previous chapters leave unexplored two chronic tensions underlying the principle of care for others. The first of these is the difference between care for (distant) others as social responsibility, sometimes expressed by the term 'social justice' and pursued as a political project, and the everyday interpersonal care in the family and community that still mostly falls to women and is seldom seen as 'work', in part because it is routinely unpaid. This care encompasses emotional as well as physical labour and, in recent history, was the private, domestic task of women. It became the template of the modern caring occupations, a fact that largely accounts for their persistently low status, poor pay and assumed lack of skill. James Butler puts it succinctly in a discussion of how 'the matrix of care work' has changed since the mid-20th century with the rise of a 'care sector' of employment in the economy of welfare and yet, at the same time, has stayed the same in spite of feminist agitation about what Daniels calls women's 'invisible' care (Daniels 1987; Butler 2023).[1] The three features that Butler believes are unchanged are the centrality of unpaid care work, its apparent invisibility, and 'its stubbornly gendered quality' (Butler 2023, p 12). Invisible, unpaid care for kin, mostly done by women, remains the default option. Even when paid care is provided and supported out of welfare spending, it supplements rather than entirely replaces its invisible counterpart.

The second tension in the principle of care is illustrated in Michael Malone's parable/novel *Handling Sin* (Malone 1984). It is a principle that has played a not inconsiderable role in the secularization of the value of care for others: the chronic contradiction between the traditional role of the institutional churches as guardians of moral standards and respectability and their Christian mission to care for all people, particularly the poor and marginalized who so often lie on the 'wrong' side of the boundary of 'respectability'. Respectability is often code for sexual conformity and/or absence of poverty or other forms of marginal status. Linda Woodhead appeals to something close to this contradiction in her 2021 Cadbury Lectures (Woodhead 2021). This chapter explores these tensions and contradictions, first by considering how they played out in the secularization debate as it focused on sex and gender.

Sex and gender in the secularization debate

A disagreement between two historians of religion about secularization in Britain, Callum Brown and Hugh McLeod, set off a long-running controversy over the role of sexuality and gender in secularization in Britain and more widely in the West. In 2001 Callum Brown published a monograph coloured by humanist and feminist ideas, *The Death of Christian Britain*. Brown argues that after a long slow decline in the 19th century, the early 1960s saw an unprecedentedly rapid abandonment of church attendance and attachment as a generation of young women rejected the traditional gender roles that had been sacralized by the Christian churches; 'the feminization of piety' was a core component of the culture of respectability. In Brown's thesis, these young 1960s women jettisoned the code of Victorian/Edwardian sexual morality and the double standard that went with it; women became the catalysts of secularization instead of the guardians of religion. The code of sexual morality that they rejected treated women's 'honour' as dependent on their sexual 'purity' – virginity up to marriage and chastity thereafter. Yet men saw it as proof of their masculinity to ignore such constraints for themselves while despising women who behaved the same way. Brown believes this produced a sexually 'repressive', normatively heterosexual culture endorsed by the churches but internalized and reproduced in the family, largely by women themselves.

Brown's novel methodological move was to show how this gender order was sustained and reinforced in popular cultural consumption – novels, short stories, magazines, biographies, autobiographies and obituaries. People learned to shape their own sense of self by transferring the model found in 'discursive Christianity' onto their own life narrative. Brown follows the French philosopher Michel Foucault, who regards 'discourse' as the locus of power that shapes individual choices to fit the requirements of the current social order: self-coercion masquerading as self-determination. The template of popular discursive Christianity is what Brown calls the 'evangelical narrative', with John Bunyan being its prime exemplar, reflecting the Christian life as a continual struggle against temptation. He identifies it in the obituaries, stories and advice columns in Christian magazines as well as in the wider popular print media.

One aspect of the 'evangelical narrative' to which Brown gives special weight is the way a 'pure' woman is called to redeem the fallen man, who may be father, brother, wooer, husband or son. This theme is hardly a core feature of Bunyan's *The Pilgrim's Progress*, but is central to early novels of the 18th and 19th centuries in the emerging genre of 'romance', with plots centred on finding a marriage partner. Brown's notion of *the* evangelical narrative is in fact a portmanteau concept with components that Brown does not always keep distinct: a perpetual struggle with temptation in which success is the path to salvation and failure is the path to degradation; a gendered difference in this struggle that, for women, principally requires the preservation of their sexual chastity but, for men, may involve a wide range of 'masculine' sins, typically involving selfishness and the pursuit of power at the expense of others or of their own personal integrity; romantic dramas of courtship leading to marriage or to disaster; and virtuous women as the 'good angels' of easily tempted men. These elements sometimes come together but are often separated in narrative, as in life. The confusion makes Brown's thesis more ambiguous than his theory acknowledges.

Although they are not the only plots in early novels – Laurence Sterne's surreal comedy *Tristram Shandy* was even more celebrated – the courtship and gender tropes and the male threats to female purity in the pioneer epistolary novels of the 18th century, such as Samuel Richardson's *Pamela* and *Clarissa*, laid the narrative foundation of the new genre of the novel. The plot of both of Richardson's tales turns on the campaign of a privileged aristocrat to seduce a virtuous woman, his young servant in *Pamela*, but a woman of his own social status in *Clarissa*. *Pamela* works like a fairy tale where the low-born servant becomes 'a lady' when her much-tried virtue is rewarded by marriage to the high-born would-be seducer. *Clarissa* is a tragedy in which both protagonists are destroyed, though not before the seducer/rapist recognizes his guilt before being killed in a duel of honour. Callum Brown regards many novels by Thackeray, Dickens, Scott and innumerable minor writers as versions of this 'evangelical' romance narrative. Certainly, many of Dickens' heroines are archetypically virtuous and modest young women – Amy Dorrit, Kate Nickleby, Esther Summerson or Agnes Whitfield could grace any evangelical narrative despite Dickens's savage, comic caricatures of evangelical clergy, while Little Em'ly is one of the tragic victims of the high-born seducer, and Thomas Hardy's Tess is another.

Brown's structuralist model is a 'discourse' composed of clusters of binary opposites – male/female, perversion/innocence, friend/enemy, selfishness/selflessness, power/powerlessness – moving the narrative through a temporal sequence from danger to victory or to tragedy. Although the examples that Brown uses mostly have an evangelical provenance, he recognizes that the whole diffused culture of reading in the Victorian age followed much the same model. That was how it became a taken-for-granted pattern of narrative expectation which remains with us in modern media including film, television, plays, musicals, and popular and literary fiction. This is true even where the model is subverted through irony, inversion or disruption, as it is, to comic effect, in Sheridan's depiction, in his play *The Rivals*, of the novel-addicted Lydia Languish.[2] Subversive moves would lose their effect if the model did not remain so familiar. The comedy and pathos of stories that never deliver the mandated 'happy ending' nor anything so dramatic as tragedy is the key to Barbara Pym's once-popular novels of failed 'romance', although the evangelical sexual moral code has as little traction in a Pym novel as it had in her own life.[3]

Brown believes that the gender order of the evangelical narrative was rejected by young women in the 1960s. They walked away from the feminization of piety, and from Christianity with it, triggering the rapid secularization that he dates from the early 1960s. Despite some sharp criticism, Brown has reiterated his thesis in subtly mutating forms. In a symposium from 2013, structured around his debate with Hugh McLeod, he summarizes, rather circumspectly: 'Christendom collapsed because most women opted to live their lives in new demographic ways and because many of them constructed their lives without religion' (Brown 2013, p 55; see also Brown 2016, 2017). By 2019, in *The Battle for Christian Britain*, Brown has broadened his thesis to embrace 'deviance' of all kinds, including sexual and religious varieties, as having 'defeated' the presumption of Christian 'normativity' (Brown 2019, p 295).

Hugh McLeod's criticisms begin with Brown's chronology: churchgoing did not begin its rapid decline until the later 1960s and was, anyway, less precipitous than Brown claims. Even then, it predated 'second wave feminism' by nearly a decade (McLeod 2005, 2007, 2013). McLeod cites a series of changes, beginning with the impact of increased affluence and going on to five other contributory changes: the decline, starting in the 1950s, of ideological subcultures dating from the 19th century, including those based on class (see Kenan Malik's related thesis); the theological radicalization that began in the early1960s (see Chapter 2); the 'sexual revolution' gathering pace from the mid-1960s; the political radicalization from the mid to late 1960s, initially heavily focused on opposition to the Vietnam War; and (only finally) women's search for greater freedom, independence and self-fulfilment. It is significant that McLeod treats the sexual revolution quite separately in both its focus and its timing from women's search for autonomy and independence. Other scholars have largely agreed with McLeod and, for example, cite evidence of significant liberalization of sexual and social values in the still-churchgoing 1950s (Christie and Gavreau 2013). Two women contributors to the symposium on the Brown/McLeod debate use evidence from autobiographies of members of the British Women's Liberation Movement. Lynn Abrams finds that respectability and religion had been decisively separated for her subjects before the 1960s (Abrams 2013), and Sandra Browne shows that women in the Women's Liberation Movement had usually rejected religion before becoming feminists, but she also recognizes significant continuities between religion and feminist ideas, notably (echoing the radical theologians) that this unsatisfactory world needs radical transformation (Browne 2013). Browne insists that the 'moral litmus test' for feminists, including religious feminists, is the rejection of 'patriarchy' in all its forms, from the church to the family: the revolution in sexual morality is a necessary implication of the principle of gender equality.

The main thrust of the criticism of Callum Brown's thesis by Hugh McLeod and others is that Brown was wrong to fuse religion and respectability, religion and sexual morality too closely, that his chronology of secularization is mistimed, and that many other social changes, such as increased affluence, mobility and individualism, were caught up in the process. The gender changes that Brown highlights did undoubtedly happen, but not in the tight harness or the simple causal chain his thesis claims. The eloquent memoir written by the journalist Deborah Orr just before her early death in 2019 shows that religion and respectability were already separated in the Scottish working-class housing estate in Motherwell where she grew up. The tyranny of respectability had certainly operated in her family from the time of her parents' youth in the early 1960s into the 1980s of her own girlhood, even though active churchgoing and belief never played any part in their life. In an obvious secular echo of the evangelical code, her unbelieving, lapsed Presbyterian father was frustrated by his glamorous wife's distaste for sex which, nevertheless, confirmed his view that she was the ideal woman. Orr writes: 'Even though religious belief was on the wane, people like my parents seemed to cling to the moral framework of the religion they'd rejected all the more' (Orr 2020, p 207).

Deborah Orr also describes sectarian division in the housing estate and schools of Motherwell as similarly detached from religious belief and church attendance – more tribal than religious. Billy Connolly, who mercilessly satirized sectarianism in his comedy routines, remembers the same disconnection in the Glasgow tenements, schools and football stadiums of his own youth in the 1970s (Connolly 2020). The persistence of sectarian identity in mainland Britain owes little to active belief or churchgoing in spite of its 'religious' labels. Both the gender order and ascribed sectarian identity are sustained by processes and discourses that can, and often do, dispense with substantive religious commitment. This means they are not automatically cancelled by secular cultural change. This paradox may well lurk in the background of identity politics in the 21st century.

Brown and McLeod, in common with most observers, agree that what moved the attitudes and expectations of women about sex and reproduction closer to those of men was the involvement of women in paid work and their access to reliable contraception under their own control and to legal, safe abortion. Yet most evidence suggests that young unmarried women's access to reliable contraception was far from complete even in the 1980s, long after attitudes and expectations as well as sexual behaviour had been transformed.[4] Certainly, changes in sexual attitudes eroded those aspects of the feminization of piety that had tied religious piety to sexual 'purity', yet the severing of that link did not cancel the assumption that women were responsible for the vast bulk of caring for others. It is clear too that much of the change in women's attitudes and expectations about sex had already begun by the 1950s (or even the 1940s), well before churchgoing and religious identity began serious decline and long before women gained effective control of their fertility – for instance, the contraceptive pill, although available from the beginning of the 1960s, was not offered to unmarried women by the NHS, or even in all private clinics, until the end of the decade; when I married in 1962, like other married women I had to have my husband's written permission to get contraception from an NHS clinic. Moreover, changes in attitudes had affected perspectives inside the churches well before the official positions of church hierarchies altered on such issues as divorce, contraception, homosexuality and sex before and within marriage. There seems to have been an unstable and patchy transition from the 1950s until at least the early 1990s before all the changes affecting women and sexuality moved into line. It was only in the 21st century that the full consequences of the sexual revolution made themselves clear.

The rejection of the feminization of piety may not have been *the* cause of the acceleration of secularization from the 1960s onwards, yet the cultural history of the concept raises issues barely addressed by Callum Brown, whose preoccupations with specifically *sexual* liberation and the rise of unbelief obscure the issues of care entangled in the gender code of the feminization of piety. The moral requirement for the sexual 'purity' of women was far more easily dislodged in British culture and patterns of behaviour than were assumptions about the gendered nature of care. Women, however sexually liberated, are still expected (and mostly expect themselves) to take primary responsibility for interpersonal care, particularly caring for their own and often other people's children (not least in the increasing numbers of complex or 'reconstituted' families in an age of unstable partnerships) and for the needy in the family and community. It is clear, for instance, that throughout the pandemic lockdowns in 2020–21, the large majority of the increased domestic work and much of the responsibility for supervising and home schooling children, fell on women and had a more negative impact on them than on men (Office for National Statistics 2021). If women did not take care of these things, major changes to the operation of the economy and the welfare services would be needed to cover all the care and maintenance that never appears as part of the nation's productivity calculations.

Revisionist feminist critiques

In *Sex and Secularism*, the American feminist historian Joan Wallach Scott, takes a Marxist feminist approach to the gender inequalities in capitalist societies, focusing on 'reproductive labour' (Scott 2018). Scott is as indebted as Callum Brown to Foucault's theory but is notably less triumphalist about the consequences for women of the Western sexual revolution. I have reservations about some aspects of her overall argument, which I shall address in due course, but her analysis opens up a little-considered aspect of how, for all the dramatic changes in religion and sexuality, women still find themselves the main carers. This is the aspect of Callum Brown's argument that fails to address women's caring role as distinct from either their piety or their sexual 'freedom'. Scott argues that it was the *discourse* of secularism that structured the normative Western pattern of gender, including the heavy burden of 'reproductive labour' assigned to women under capitalism – that is, their responsibility for creating and sustaining generations of workers, a responsibility through which care is so often worked out.

Scott sees secularism as a fluid, polemical term rather than a universally applicable abstraction or an empirical description of institutions and politics. For Scott, secularism is a 'discourse ... put to work differently in different contexts'. It rhetorically positions itself as a feature of 'modernity' and identifies as its enemy whatever is seen as its opposite (Scott 2018, p 183). Scott argues that what matters about concepts such as 'gender', 'sex', 'freedom' or 'secularity' is not what they *universally* signify but what work the appeal to them is made to do within the discourse of secularism in historically specific contexts. She maintains that gender and politics have been 'mutually constitutive' in capitalist societies. This is because gender and power are both inherently unstable constructs, always challengeable and insecure as the rationale for asymmetrical or unequal relationships in any particular context. Gender and power each appeal to the other's supposed timeless and immutable character to mirror and shore up its own.

Scott describes 19th-century secularism as an anticlerical discourse in America, Britain and Europe that successfully eclipsed/incorporated/superseded the Christian biblical justification of gender asymmetry by using 'rational', 'scientific' claims about what was 'natural' to each sex. She traces the mutation of the gender order of 'separate and unequal' roles and status for males and females in capitalist reproductive labour from its earlier biblical justification as the divine creation through its 'reinscription' into modern biological science. Woman's role as carer is justified by her biological nature rather than by divine fiat. Scott tracks women's eventual entry into the male political sphere of politics, showing that entry does not mean equality. The Victorian binary that assigned the 'public sphere' to men and the 'private sphere' to women had eventually enabled women to extend their 'private' 'domestic' concerns into the 'social' realm, encompassing such things as family, children, hygiene and welfare. This incursion acted as a conduit for women's entry into the 'public' sphere of politics which culminated in female suffrage. The vote, however did not bring women equality of power. The public sphere of masculine power, focused in the state and the economy, kept and still retains its domination. The state concerned itself with the market rather than the lesser arena of social welfare, which it largely left to women, the churches and charity. This pattern, by which the capitalist state treats economic matters as primary while welfare issues are secondary, remains essentially intact in the 21st century. Scott's argument that welfare still retains much of its earlier 'private' meaning even after being transferred to the political arena of the state is more than plausible even where capitalism is politically modified by other social values as it is in 'welfare' states. This argument that the public/private binary echoes and continues an older male/female one is clearly implicated in the continuing lowly status of care and the care sector.

Scott further argues that the historical mutation of gender within the discourse of secularism as contemporary Western 'sexual emancipation', simply lays a further burden on women but represents it as a self-chosen 'freedom'. The construction of female sexuality shifts from exclusively serving reproduction in the family to becoming the contemporary liberation of what she terms the 'uncovered', desiring, female body, engaging in 'autonomous, self-willed, individual action' and open to 'a diversity of sexual practices' (Scott 2018, p 181). Yet, she comments:

> this vision of sexual emancipation is not a realization of a universal freedom but is instead a historically specific creation: a Western middle-class notion of what it means to be free. It is, moreover, a freedom that does not necessarily confer equality – the asymmetry of the difference of sex continues both in the most intimate of relationships as well as in the marketplace of jobs and ideas.

Scott believes that liberated sexuality in the West does not bring equality except in subjecting desiring bodies, male and female alike, to market logic, making them 'at once consumers and commodities' (Scott 2018, p 177).

Scott claims, almost in passing, that '[t]here is … a persistent Christian dimension in this discourse [of secularism]' (Scott 2018, p 182). Yet she never fully explains precisely what this is. Another unsatisfactory aspect of her argument is that although she describes successive changes in the content and context of the 'fluid' discourse of secularity, she seldom examines in much historical detail the how and why of these shifts, being mainly concerned to establish the unchanging co-constitution of gender inequalities and power in the discourse. Citing the 'reinscription' of gender asymmetry from the Bible onto science is not a full explanation of the process of 'collusion' that she claims. Moreover, while asymmetries of power are the subject of her analysis, she tends to treat both power and capitalism as abstractions even though she is highly critical of the use of reifying abstractions.

She concludes her book with an account of the way the political/rhetorical role assigned to Islam in the 21st-century secularist discourse of the West, especially in the US, is as the prime contemporary enemy of 'freedom'. This is despite the US's own persistent culture wars over gender that pit 'fundamentalist' Christians against 'enlightened' opinion in a way that might appear to qualify 'Christians' as the more obvious 'enemy' in the secularist discourse. Yet Scott claims it is the 'covered' body of the obedient Muslim woman that is fantasized as the 'antithesis of whatever "equality" means in the West', as 'abject' and deprived of individual agency by male domination, and then presented as the religious enemy of secularism. Fundamentalist Christians in the US are not representative of the wide variety of Western Christianity, and Scott never satisfactorily specifies the historical or contemporary role Christianity plays in the discourse of secularism and its identification of Islam as the enemy. Nevertheless, her indictment of the new gender inequalities in the secularist discourse of Western sexual 'freedom' are an instructive historical feature of the history of the feminization of piety. They are, one might think, the latest, onerous addition to the duty of care that women owe to men while being represented as what women owe to themselves.

What has been referred to as a new wave of 'Puritan' or 'reactionary' feminism amplifies Scott's critique, particularly on the asymmetries that mark 'liberated' sexual power. For instance, Louise Perry argues that the sexual revolution has been uniquely damaging to women and children (Perry 2022). Technological advances in contraception and the availability of legal abortion make it plausible for women to be represented as idealized 'liberal subjects', autonomous and indistinguishable from men in their ability to 'choose' and enjoy sexual promiscuity without consequences. Some second wave feminists had arrived at a similar conclusion about the downside for women of mass contraception when they complained about men in various progressive political groups in the late 1960s who confined women to backroom roles and expected them to make the coffee and be sexually available.[5] Perry, like Scott, believes this is a distinctively masculine model of the bourgeois 'liberal subject' and that it is exploitative in expecting women's desires to conform to those of men. Male desires are increasingly shaped by early exposure to pornography that typically exaggerates precisely those stereotypes of sexual difference so derided by second wave feminists as damaging and coercive social constructs. Men and women today are expected to be equally 'uninhibited', but women's desires are now required to encompass humiliation and violence from men. These expectations load on to women a new duty to use a mixture of dieting and cosmetic surgery to sculp their bodies to meet pornographic ideals, much as the women 'influencers' in the Kardashian family in America have done. Perry believes that contemporary sexual culture, particularly in today's unregulated digital media, ignores the role of specifically female reproductive capacities in the constitution of female desire, including the time limit on female fertility. A realistic 'informed consent' cannot happen without recognizing this difference. Perry echoes Scott's view of the 'commodification' of desire and the desiring body.

Mary Harrington's analysis is even darker. *Feminism against Progress* (Harrington 2023) is a notably fierce polemic against the sexual revolution from the standpoint of what she calls 'reactionary feminism'. Her argument is the fruit of an epiphany she had after living the first part of her adult life in what she belatedly recognized as the dystopia of the sexual revolution, in which, in common with Louise Perry, she found the old sexual double standard masquerading as 'freedom' and inducing women to contort female sexual desire to meet the market norm of a pornographic male model of uncommitted sexual 'pleasure'. Harrington argues that the changes lauded as the achievement of 'progress' have actually commodified ever more aspects of our sexual lives. What she refers to as the (secular) 'Theology of Progress', which motivated the quest for sexual freedom and self-realization by second wave feminism, in reality was the product of industrialized technology applied to sexual life. Contraception renders adult women 'sterile as the default state'; digital communication services a market in supposedly cost-free sexual hook-ups; and medical and therapeutic technology promises to erase the limits that biology imposes on individual freedom of choice through what Harrington memorably calls 'Meat Lego Gnosticism' – medical, psychological and technological reshaping with the aim of transcending the 'lumbering flesh' with which we are each encumbered from birth. The effects of all this have been to alienate men and women from each other and humans in general from 'nature', including our own inescapably embodied human nature. In Mary Harrington's own case, liberation from that bleak 'freedom' came through choosing heterosexual marriage and motherhood with all their constraints, necessary elements of self-denial, hard efforts of cooperation and lasting satisfactions. Harrington's conclusion is that we, men and women, need to embrace the inevitability and blessings of embodiment, of limits and commitment, to reclaim our natural bodies, including biological sexual difference, to take back the privilege of caring directly for our children rather than subcontracting it to others, and recognizing the need for sexual partners and parents to work together and nurture each other and their children. Her disillusionment with the industrialized technologies shaping human sex lives seems to have driven her to condemn the hormonal roller-coaster and 'unnaturalness' of chemical contraception as worse for women than reconnecting sex to the risk of pregnancy, and it has left her with deep repugnance for abortion. She concedes that the 'old rules' that had shielded women and children from the worst effects of the 'unprotected' sex she is now advocating are no longer in place, but she does not suggest how to replace them. Nor does she consider that a similarly literal return to unmodified 'nature' would leave us without antibiotics and the other blessings of modern medicine that clearly saved her life and the life of her daughter when the birth ran into problems. Perhaps so deep a personal dive into the sexual revolution was traumatic enough to excuse what may be rhetorical hyperbole. The destruction of the moral and psychological primacy of care, as much as the impoverishment of desire, is at the heart of her 'reactionary' conversion. She writes:

> as women, we have joined men in embracing the Rousseauean vision of autonomous personhood, and rejecting caring obligations as an obstacle to self-realisation, so in turn care has been institutionalised, proceduralised and depersonalised – all the way down to infancy. In the wake of this shift, a generation has grown up that regards the suffocating 'care' of a risk-averse, third-party pseudo-parent not as the enemy of their individual flourishing, but as its enabling condition. (Harrington 2023, p 127)

Mary Harrington is a member of the millennial generation, which has seen the full negative experience of the 'sexual revolution'. It is not yet clear how many among subsequent generations will follow her in her radical disillusion. Something like the ideal of casual sex without 'catching feelings' or entailing consequences is prominent among Gen Z, although mainly, perhaps, as a time-limited stage of extended pre-maturity before finding a secure place in the labour market, entering a committed partnership and founding a family, an aspiration that seems not yet a complete anachronism (Katz et al 2021). Louise Perry and Mary Harrington largely ignore religion in their analyses, but both insist, as Scott does, how inimical the culture of liberated sex is to the values of nurture and commitment, without which children do not thrive. Mary Harrington believes that being alienated from the *natural* desire to care for others is the worst impoverishment women have imposed on themselves in the name of progress. The sexual revolution has sharply separated sexual pleasure from the value of care for others or, in extreme cases, even care for the self. In this unillusioned view, liberated sexuality is not the unproblematic secular triumph for women that Callum Brown celebrates.

The back history of the feminization of piety

The history of the feminization of piety (which is itself a 'mutating discourse' in Scott's terms) may shed some light on any collusions between Christianity and secularist discourse indicated by Scott (2018), and perhaps provide clues to the persistence of the assumption that caring is primarily women's responsibility even after women have become a significant part of the paid labour market and 'liberated' sexual beings. I begin my exploration with the curious fact that, after many centuries of having been the sex that in the biblical creation myth caused the Fall when Eve offered the forbidden apple to Adam, around the end of the 18th century women somehow came to be represented as the pious sex rather than Eve's temptress daughters requiring the steady controlling hand of moral men. This reminds us that the gender order is subject to periodic change and that other patterns predate the feminization of piety, and there may well be further variants in the making that even Mary Harrington has not anticipated. The historical inversion of the attribution of blame between Adam and Eve in the late 18th century may well be one of the points at which changes in how Christianity was lived, contributed to, or colluded with an incipient discourse of secularism.

Celibacy had spiritual priority from Christianity's earliest years when the Second Coming was expected imminently. In the meantime, spiritual families of brothers and sisters in Christ, in principle, took precedence over the claims of blood kin and patriarchal family systems. Both had long-standing consequences for Christian societies, including exclusive male leadership in church and society, the idealization of virginity and placing obligations to the Christian church and community before loyalty to family and kin; for centuries that provided escape routes for some 'pious' women from the burden of kinship demands. The Protestant Reformation spiritually demoted monasticism and celibacy and, in a clear secularizing move, made everyday life, including marriage and family, the proper arena of salvation. Henry VIII in England was not only responsible for the dissolution of the monasteries but as head of the English church he acquiesced in reducing the church's seven sacraments to two, baptism and the Eucharist, in accordance with the policy of the Reformers. He had wanted to declare marriage a sacrament to underline the demotion of monasticism, but this contradicted the Protestant Reformers. Henry was dissuaded by Cranmer, and in the Book of Common Prayer the compromise was to call the marriage service 'The Solemnisation of Matrimony'.[6] In the 17th century, Milton made a Protestant case for divorce, defending the importance of intellectual and spiritual compatibility between spouses. By the early 18th century, the passionate High Anglican ascetic Mary Astell was able to publish something very close to Milton's Reforming argument but from a High Tory and 'enlightened' viewpoint, including a plea for equal access to education so that women could exercise rational choice about whether or whom to marry. Gender was entering public conversation in new ways, not least in various combinations of Christian and Enlightenment ideas that were concerned with improving the working of society by the application of a combination of rational and moral principles.

A new discourse of 'feminization'

From the late 17th century in the American colonies, and from the early 18th century in Britain and Europe, more women than men attended church services. This partly reflected demographic change, but also marked increased lay male reluctance to attend worship, instead regarding their womenfolk as their deputies in religious matters. At the same time, the rise of a commercial economy altered thinking about economic behaviour and women's role in it. Lucy Delap, notes the common fear in North America and Europe that women's 'perceived love of luxury and gossip' might threaten economic progress and therefore required rational education for women as a corrective (Delap 2020, p 60 et seq). Max Weber famously argued that early Calvinism had been the engine of early capitalism, partly through its rigorous emphasis on frugality and self-denial, the 'Protestant Ethic', which had the effect, fortunate for capitalist development, of encouraging entrepreneurial capital accumulation. The developing commercial economy of the 19th century, however, seemed increasingly to call for a different 'spirit' that would encourage consumption.

An emerging breed of political economists offered a rough moral solution by arguing that individually selfish choices worked to the good of the whole (*pace* Adam Smith's emphasis on moral sentiments as one of the necessary underpinnings of the rules of economic life). Yet gender had no (acknowledged) part in their models of *Homo economicus*. In an argument that parallels Lucy Delap's observation, E. J. Clery identifies middle-class women's patterns of consumption as the fulcrum of a change that started a 'feminization debate' in the late 18th century which radiated into many spheres of life. The debate was conducted through journalism, essays, popular prints and engravings such as those of Hogarth, satires like those of Swift and Pope, and the new genre of novels by Richardson, Defoe and Smollett (Clery 2004). Women were reading the novels but the debates were the province of men, conducted in the new coffee houses and men's clubs. The argument centred on the way the wives and daughters of the emerging business and professional classes were reforming morals and manners in the home, elevating aesthetic as well as ethical and religious standards. The new consumer commodities – food, homewares, furnishing and fashion – were the props and stage sets of the increasingly refined dramas of polite life that supplied the stuff of imaginative fiction, theatre and poetry. In

France the new ideas radiated out from the salons of aristocratic women, attended by influential male intellectuals: in a few cases, all-women salons emerged as an early 'feminist' initiative (Delap 2020, p 101 et seq; Scott 2018, pp 80, 104). In Britain the diffusion of the new 'civilized' culture of manners and morals mostly operated informally though the homes of the rising professional and business classes and the new arenas of public debate and opinion formation.

The feminization argument challenged the view that consumer luxuries were effeminizing and corrupting a manly, austere Britain, which depended on now-threatened virile and ascetic virtues to build the flourishing commercial economy of the British Empire. Clery shows how the debate engaged reformers of many kinds, encompassing evangelicals, political economists and political actors. It occurred within a discourse she calls 'civic humanism', based on classical Greek and Roman models of the (exclusively male) republican warrior-citizen. She writes: 'a discourse of feminization came to challenge the masculinist paradigm that had shaped [civic humanism]' (Clery 2004, p 6). Reformers abandoned the cyclical model of history in the Greek and Roman classics in favour of the linear model taken from Christianity and transplanted to the Enlightenment belief in 'progress'.

The new salience of gender took many forms. The Romantic movement gave an importance to emotion, which, through its association with female sensibility, had been deemed inferior to 'masculine' reason and calculation even by Enlightenment writers, notably Rousseau. The evangelical movement turned this into the feminization of piety. Lutheran Pietism in Germany was a link between the two movements, exemplified in the poetry of Novalis or the nature poetry and religious librettos of Barthold Heinrich Brockes.[7] In Britain the 'experimental' or 'experiential' religion of the evangelical revival was powerfully represented by the Wesley brothers and the Methodist movement they led, John through his preaching, and Charles through his hymns. Both brothers were considerable theologians but were popularly characterized by the emotionality of their faith, even though John Wesley often deplored the dangers of emotional excess, especially among women. Although there are clear parallels with the Ignatian spirituality of post-Reformation Catholicism, in the 18th-century Protestant world a religion of personal feeling was seen as quintessentially feminine, even effeminate when taken up by men, especially priests and ministers of the church.

In a celebrated feminist book, Ann Douglas argued that in 19th-century America, the decline of religion among men led women and clergy to try to influence the only arena open to them, the arts and literature (Douglas 1977). Douglas believes they wrote books idealizing the qualities that kept them powerless – timidity, piety and disdain for competition – which she calls 'sentimental' values. This chimes with Callum Brown's depiction of the 'discourse' of the evangelical narrative. Both Douglas and Brown regard the reversal of the moral status of men and women as complete by 1800. In the 19th century, men became the morally fragile sex, whose very masculinity predisposed them to violence and made them competitive and physical in ways that opened them to temptation.

Public/private, male/female binaries

Economic change and the growth of urban areas had created conditions in which a significant sector of the new business and professional classes could copy the aristocracy in keeping their wives and daughters out of the world of employment and turn the domestic arena into women's sphere. This was not true for the labouring classes, whose women had always done as much physical and 'manual' labour as the men (Griffin 2020). Nevertheless it became the accepted ideal for women and men to keep to their own proper sphere. As Scott notes, men were assigned the public sphere of work and politics, commerce and intellectual endeavour (Scott 2018). Women were assigned the domestic world of homemaking, child rearing and family care, including the religious formation of children, their early education, and keeping men on the right moral and religious path while remaining submissive to male authority. It was a highly moralized biblical ideal of womanhood that later tended to assume that the female caring role was built into women's genetic make-up as biologically 'natural'. It became taken for granted that women were the carers in all social classes and, as Virginia Woolf frequently complained, 'the angel in the house', like her mother Julia Stephen, who at the turn of the 19th to the 20th century not only cared for the children of her two marriages but took charity and comforts to the poor, even though the Stephen household was notoriously irreligious (Lee 2007; Light 2008). We see the gender order, again, having a life beyond religious justification.

'The angel in the house' and her critics

'The angel in the house' is the title of a poem, published in a sequence of three by Coventry Patmore between 1854 and 1862. The phrase came to be used as shorthand for the saintly domestic woman by both admirers and critics of the gender order it represented (Hogan and Bradstock 1998). At virtually the same time as Coventry Patmore's 'sentimental' poems, in 1856 Elizabeth Barrett Browning published her most significant late work, the verse novel *Aurora Leigh*, a passionate rebuke to the ideal of 'the angel in the house' (Barrett-Browning nd). It was, nevertheless, admired by Coventry Patmore himself along with many other male writers, including Ruskin and Tennyson, and also by women writers such as Emily Dickinson, whom it inspired, and George Eliot, who saw it as a powerful vindication of the sensibilities of women writers like the fictional Aurora, as well as Mary Ann Evans and Elizabeth Barrett Browning themselves, who, no less than men, strove for 'ample being' (Sampson 2021, p 235).

Aurora Leigh was a bestseller, and its success makes clear that even in the high Victorian age Callum Brown's evangelical narrative did not quite sweep all before it. Aurora Leigh rejects her cousin Romney, the man she loves, and who loves her, because he 'Supposed me a thing too small, to deign to know' (Sampson 2021, p 234). He wants her for a wife who will be his meek and supportive helpmeet in *his* work of social reform. She chooses instead to be a poet. After the melodramatic climax of the subplot, the two only come together when, like Mr Rochester in *Jane Eyre*, Romney is blinded in a fire, and finally able to 'see' Aurora's strength of purpose and her success as a published poet not as unwomanly but as strong and admirable. The convoluted subplot concerns Marian Erle, Aurora's protégée and Romney's second-choice fiancée, whose rape is engineered by Lady Waldemar, who wants to marry Romney herself. Marian valiantly chooses to raise her son in defiance of the shame and condemnation that was the expected fate of the 'fallen woman'. Defying the mores of the time, Marian is the second heroine of the poem.

Elizabeth Barrett Browning was surprised by the success of *Aurora Leigh* when she had feared she would be 'put in the stocks and pelted with the eggs of the last twenty years' singing birds as a disorderly woman and free-thinking poet' (Sampson 2021, p 235). She was not a 'free thinker' in the terms of the time but, following her husband, Robert, was abreast of the latest biblical criticism and shared Robert's Dissenting conviction that believers should think for themselves. She was also one of the heirs in a wealthy family of sugar traders with slave estates in the Caribbean. Financial independence and marriage to a penniless fellow poet were both made possible by her share in that tainted inheritance, which finally allowed her to distance herself from some of her father's values. She became a passionate abolitionist and, even after having a son, never repudiated her opinion that conventional caring roles for women were 'retrograde – a revival of old virtues', 'not the best use to which we can put a gifted and accomplished woman' (Sampson 2021, p 231). Yet, like Virginia Woolf two generations later, her accomplishments as a woman writer were dependent on the work of (mainly women) servants and other members of her family doing the heavy lifting of day-to-day care (Light 2008, pp 75–159).

Virginia Woolf vehemently rejected the tradition of women taking care of others as it applied to herself and other women writers and artists, but at the same time she clung to it when it came to her own desire to be cared for. Woolf's biographer, Hermione Lee, describes Woolf's lifelong ambivalence about her mother's feminine good works:

> [Julia Stephen] believed in working for good in a practical way in her immediate domestic circle and through benevolent institutions. She seems to have fully endorsed the Victorian models for female behaviour, as found in Dickens' Esther in *Bleak House* … or – come to that – in Coventry Patmore's *Angel in the House* … Virginia Woolf spent much of her writing life exposing and analysing those roles, but also in looking longingly back to the world which engendered them. There is an extraordinary gap between her satirical repudiation of acceptable behaviour for women in *Three Guineas* or *The Years* and the affectionate yearning with which she recalls the culture of her mother's generation. (Lee 1997, p 85)

Alison Light comments on Woolf's simultaneous resentment of the intrusion of (female) servants into her privacy and her demand that they 'took turns at playing mother and child' (Light 2008, p 173). A similar ambivalence about women as nurturers surfaces again among some of the women's liberationists of the 1960s and 1970s who were intent on deconstructing morally coercive elements of the female role, as we shall see in a later chapter.

Elizabeth Barrett Browning, the privileged invalid, both resisted and acquiesced in her gender role, taking whichever stance most effectively protected her independence as a poet (Sampson 2021). She was not alone in such ambivalent resistance. Around the time *Aurora Leigh* appeared, there was a popular cult of opera, with travelling companies finding large enthusiastic audiences in Britain's provincial cities, including substantial numbers of the working class, many of them women. The favourites were Verdi's *La traviata*, with a courtesan heroine, Violetta, modelled on a real-life counterpart from the Paris slums, and Bizet's *Carmen*, with Carmen a seductress from a Spanish cigarette factory (Williams 2020). Heroines at this period usually pay for their 'transgressive' sexuality in operas and novels by ending the story dead (Kernan 2006; Higgins 2013). Although these operas may be at best an ambivalent defiance of the prevalent gender order, they revel in the 'unthinkable' that respectable women were expected to look away from. Despite this undertow of dissent, the unequal Victorian gender order was largely sustained until the eve of the First World War before meeting increasing resistance.

Muscular Christianity: an evangelical response to the 'feminization' discourse

In the mid-19th century, a sector of the churches had found the evangelical focus on a religion of feeling 'emasculating'. 'Muscular Christianity' asserted the manly, heroic aspects of sustaining and spreading the faith and encouraging physical fitness, the virtues that it was believed had expanded the mission field and sustained the British Empire; in effect, a 'Christianization' of the 'classical' virtues of what Emma Clery (2004, p 6) refers to as 'civic humanism'. Muscular Christianity was widely adopted by the new public schools educating the sons of the elite alongside those of the rising commercial classes. It found notable expression in the work of Charles Kingsley and Thomas Hughes, inspired associations such as the Scouts, the Church Army and the Young Men's Christian Association, and travelled the world with the 'servants of the British Empire'. It often provided the model hero of the evangelical narrative.

At the mid-century when this movement emerged, around a third of bishops in the established church were evangelicals, some of them 'muscular Christians'. Evangelicals initiated a range of social reforms, including the abolition of slavery, the improvement of morals and manners and the education of the labouring classes. Many projects were conducted by philanthropic women whose causes included keeping Sundays free from work, partly so that the lower classes could attend worship; reclaiming prostitutes and training them for 'useful work'; founding orphanages for abandoned infants and sometimes training them for domestic service, as was the case for one of Virginia Woolf's servants, Lottie Hope (Light 2008, pp 75–159, 315–44, especially p 321). This is the kind of activity that Joan Wallach Scott is referring to when she describes women taking the 'domestic' and 'private' from the home out into the public sphere in the first move making tentative inroads in the public/private binary. Evangelical ladies tutored women of the lower orders in the domestic arts, budgeting and educating their children, especially in the Christian virtues. The drawback to the programme was that many lower-class women, either through being unmarried or having lost the male breadwinner to the common tragedy of death or desertion, had to work in factories and workshops, as seamstresses, informal street sellers or, in very large numbers, as the domestic servants who took the bulk of the work in the home off the hands of their middle- and upper-class mistresses. The philanthropists' ambition to turn their working-class sisters into 'angels in the house' ran up against serious practical hurdles. What they could and did do was to spread their message through a new genre of popular literature to the newly literate masses in the industrial town. This literature is the subject of the following chapter.

5

The Popular Evangelical Narrative of Care and Some Modern Analogues

Mass literacy and the evangelical culture of care

From the early 19th century, the popular literature published as part of the mission to the urban poor in Britain was associated with the establishment of schools and Sunday schools to extend the rudiments of education and discipline along with Christianity to the children of the poor. In the late 18th century Hannah More was one of the earliest writers to target the labouring classes with a new genre of cheap publications of this sort. Initially, she disapproved of teaching the poor to read for fear of exposing them to revolutionary writings around the time of the French Revolution. When she realized that the lower orders were already reading cheap sensational fiction, More changed tack and founded schools so the children of the poor would have access to the Bible. Already a well-connected playwright, More published Cheap Repository Tracts telling simple tales with religious and political messages of loyalty, patriotism and morality of a Burkean variety. They were a success and though, at a penny, they were genuinely cheap, they eventually made profits for the publisher. It was an early sign of the publishing revolution which first provided uplifting fiction for the middle classes and then reached out to the labouring classes in harness with efforts to extend literacy to them and their children.

This was the milieu out of which the popularization of the 'evangelical narrative' of Callum Brown's (2001) theory emerged, but, in my view, more importantly, the reinforcement of a Christian culture of care. More than a hundred new periodicals appeared in the 1860s and 1870s, and some libraries added children's sections (Lang 1980). After the Education Act 1870, tracts, novels and magazines marketed to the lower orders became serious money-spinners. From the late 18th century, the practice had grown up of giving 'reward' or 'prize' books for Sunday school attendance, often with an ex-libris bookplate (Reynolds 2008). Attending Sunday school was closely associated with acquiring books in working-class homes at a time when few libraries accessible to the poor had yet opened a children's section, even though children's books were the fastest-expanding sector (Reynolds 2008). Many successful authors who published through the Religious Tract Society became mainstays of the reward book industry. The most successful of them in the mid-19th century was Hesba Stretton. Her most celebrated novel, *Jessica's First Prayer*, had sold one and a half million copies by the end of the century, ten times more than the genre-transforming *Alice* books by Lewis Carroll, which were entertainments for middle-class children rather than sources of educational, moral or religious uplift (Susina 2009, pp 95–116). Hesba Stretton was succeeded by the prolific novelist Silas Kitto Hocking as the bestselling stalwart of the prize book lists from the 1870s to the 1920s. The legacy of this popular genre to the 'feminization' of the culture of care was significant.

Prize books

Hesba Stretton was the pseudonym of Sarah Smith (1832–1911) one of four daughters of a bookseller and printer in Wellington and his Methodist wife. Sarah became a journalist and novelist, encouraged by Dickens after he published one of her early stories. She was an evangelical whose passion was social reform and the plight of the poor, particularly women and children. Silas K. Hocking (1850–1935), more than a generation younger, was brought up in Cornwall and became a Methodist minister, working in several parts of the country, including Liverpool, Manchester and London. Through his prodigious output of novels and his concern for social reform, he made friends and acquaintances in Liberal politics and in literary and publishing circles, including Conan Doyle and E.F. (Fred) Benson. He worked to increase Nonconformist influence in schools after the Education Act 1902, and after the First World War, which, as a pacifist, he found acutely distressing, he threw his efforts into work for the League of Nations. Hesba Stretton and Silas Hocking wrote the bestsellers of their times, for child and adult readers alike. In my own childhood, their novels, usually prizes for day school or Sunday school attendance, were still the only books in many working-class households in the industrial North West. They were long-lived carriers of 'the' evangelical narrative and the feminization of piety to working-class families.

These books were part of my own childhood. When I recently re-read them, I found I had forgotten many details of the plots but retained a vivid memory of their social reform message, especially the urgency of caring for others, starting in the family. Methodist Sunday school prizes were the only books, apart from the family Bible, in my paternal grandmother's house.

When I used to visit around the age of seven or eight, I would devour Hesba Stretton's *Little Meg's Children* and Silas Hocking's *Her Benny* again and again as the grown-ups talked. My daughter had a similar experience with a slightly wider selection of prize books on visits to her own (Methodist) paternal grandparents' house on Sunday afternoons in the late 1960s and early 1970s. There was a sprinkling of lesser imitators among the books, but Stretton and Hocking were the ones we both returned to. Neither my brothers nor my sons ever read these books, but they prepared me and my daughter in turn for children's novels and adult literature, just as they had led my mother-in-law to Thomas Hardy's novels in her native Dorset before she joined the army of Edwardian domestic servants in the towns and big cities. In my case, the prize books led me immediately to Kingsley's *The Water Babies*, Barrie's *Peter Pan* novels, Bunyan's *Pilgrim's Progress* and the whole addictive sequence of Louisa M. Alcott's Little Women novels – I recollect more than once sitting on the doorstep of the Co-op library waiting for it to open to find the next volume, as the rules did not allow me to take out two books in the same day – then Harriet Beecher Stowe's *Uncle Tom's Cabin* and smoothly on to Dickens, Hardy, Thackeray, Trollope, George Eliot and beyond. My daughter took in the Katy books en route to C.S. Lewis' Narnia and Tolkien's Middle-earth Alan Garnett, Peter Dickinson, Ursula Le Guin and other children's novelists of the 1960s and 1970s.[1] She had the benefit of Hesba Stretton's *Jessica's First Prayer*, which had not been in my grandmother's little collection.

My daughter also had the dubious pleasure of an unforgettable prize book, *Maggie's Mistake*, which we have been unable to track down. Maggie is a young servant whose 'mistake' is to go to a jumble sale on her Sunday afternoon off duty instead of attending chapel. In her absence, the Big House is burgled and Maggie is assumed to be the 'insider' who let in the thieves. She is dismissed and finds herself unemployable and starving in a city slum, consoled on her deathbed only by the news that the real culprit has been caught. My daughter was so outraged by this tale of grossly disproportionate human and divine retribution that she has never forgotten it – a clear case of overkill undermining evangelical intention, at least for a modern child. Yet it is worth recalling the history of my father-in-law. He had been an adolescent convert of the British evangelist Rodney 'Gypsy' Smith in the early 20th century. My father-in-law grew up in a rural labouring family in Hertfordshire with an illiterate mother and an alcoholic, though later similarly converted, father. To the end of his long life, this lovable, teetotal, revivalist street preacher had nothing troubling his conscience except a single misdemeanour as a young chauffeur before the First World War. Without asking permission, he drove his employer's precious Delaunay Bellville to visit his mother on his afternoon off duty. It did not assuage his guilt towards the end of his life over seventy years later that he had never been found out.

The moral code of Edwardian 'service' must have been every bit as fierce in his eyes as it was in *Maggie's Mistake*.

The novels by Hesba Stretton and Silas Hocking are part of a genre known as 'street Arab' or 'outcast' tales that were essentially invented by Stretton in the 1840s and then widely copied. The term persisted in the half-affectionate scolding common in my childhood when muddy or dishevelled children, usually boys, were called 'dirty little Arabs' (Lomax 2008). The 'street Arab' genre of stories was initially aimed by the publishers at the 'servant class market', but increasingly sold as part of the extension of child literature, often for children to read to their illiterate parents. In a book on Lewis Carroll, Jan Susina, sees a connection to the 'street Arab' genre in the caption of a photograph by Charles Dodgson of 'Alice Liddell as a beggar-maid' (Susina 2009, pp 95–107).[2] Hesba Stretton's concern with social reform was what had attracted the attention and support of Dickens. Elaine Lomax argues that she saw the women of the poor districts of industrial towns as having collective experiences and shared grievances, with mothers as the first casualties of poverty; the slum environment drove destitute women to drink, as it still can (Lomax 2008). In Stretton's two Jessica novels, Jessica's mother, an alcoholic, irregularly employed 'actress' in the West End of London, neglects and then abandons her little daughter. Stretton paints an unsentimental picture of alcoholism as a reaction to the poverty and hopelessness of an unsupported mother. Jessica's mother drowns herself in the Thames at the climax of *Jessica's Mother*, which may be less a melodramatic cliché of sensational fiction than a simple reflection of an everyday reality in Victorian London as almost the only affordable method of suicide for destitute women, as unsupported and unemployable mothers so often were (Stretton 1865, 1904).[3] Stretton believed the rights of mothers and children were always entwined and that women in general and mothers in particular were a humanizing influence in society; Stretton's first description of Meg in *Little Meg's Children* as a 'stunted' child 'of London growth' wearing 'the shrewd, anxious look of a woman … who was already weary with much labour' shows Stretton's sense of that visceral connection between the plight of women and children among the poor (Stretton 1868, pp 9–10). Lomax (2008) discusses one of Stretton's later novels, *Under the Old Roof*, written around the time of the amendment of the Married Women's Property Act 1870. It is a pungent tale showing a woman as no more than the legal slave and property of a man. Stretton herself remained unmarried and, thanks to an enlightened father and brother, always controlled her own earnings.

From the beginning, writers employed the evangelical narrative for several distinct purposes. Hannah More used her tales to inculcate patriotism and anti-revolutionary sentiments among the poor. Several decades later, Hesba Stretton used the same genre, in Elaine Lomax's words, 'as a vehicle for social and political projects' that 'challenged the state' with radical and even 'pro-feminist' sentiments (Lomax 2008, p 144; see also Lomax 2009). Stretton's novels were sometimes sensationalist and certainly carried an evangelical religious message but always as applied to real social injustices. They pleaded many social causes and were conspicuously concerned with the state of poor, abandoned and exploited children, the plight of young criminals, streetwalkers, street children and the abuse of domestic servants. Stretton supported Dr Barnardo's work for street children and in 1884 was a founding member of the Society for the Prevention of Cruelty to Children (now the National Society for the Prevention of Cruelty to Children) and was a member of its executive for the next decade. When she died in 1911 the total sales of her books exceeded £2 million and were the commercial lifeline of the Religious Tract Society.

Her successor, Silas Hocking, wrote short novels that appeared at a rate of one a year from the 1870s to the 1920s and advanced a reform programme and a Christian pacifist message – he opposed the Boer War, as he later opposed the First World War. The son of a Cornish tin mine owner, he had been ordained minister as a very young man in a notably democratic offshoot of Wesleyanism, the United Methodist Free Church. In 1873 his circuit was in Liverpool and he worked close to the docks, the setting of his second and most successful novel, *Her Benny*. It was first published in the United Methodist Church magazine before being taken up by Warne publishers in 1874: Warne paid Hocking £10 for what proved to be a publishing windfall for them. By the 1890s, *Her Benny* had sold a million copies, and in the 1920s it was made into a silent film. In the 1880s, Hocking moved to the City Mission in Manchester, where he worked with prostitutes and observed, as Hesba Stretton had, how poverty trapped lower-class women between terrible alternatives. In 1901, Arnold Bennett, not yet the successful novelist he was to become, noted with a touch of envy that for twenty years Silas Hocking's novels had sold at a rate of 1,000 copies a week (Bennett 1901, p 145).

Sexual sin and care for others in popular prize novels

Little Meg's Children

When I read these novels as a child, their sexual moral totally escaped me, though it was there, usually in the figure of the 'fallen woman'. What came through unforgettably was the imperative of caring for others, beginning in the family. In *Little Meg's Children*, Meg, at perhaps ten years old, is the only person left to take care of her little brother and the sickly baby when her mother dies while her father is at sea. They live in a bare room in a London slum courtyard near the docks, and Meg has to manage everything until her father returns, including her mother's funeral and then that of the baby. Money soon runs out and she pawns anything that can be spared, including her only decent dress. Kitty, the young woman in the next room, has just been released from prison and is ostracized by the neighbours. Kitty helps Meg because Meg's mother was the only person who ever spoke kindly to her; she was 'the angel in the house' who flouted respectability by speaking to the outcast Kitty. The other kindness Meg meets comes from the motherly woman at the bakery, Mrs Blossom, who gives Meg more than her little money really buys. Kitty bewails her own 'badness', especially when she sees the little family at prayer, and sometimes disappears and returns drunk. Yet she bargains with the pawnbroker on Meg's behalf and inquires at the docks why her father's ship has not docked when it was expected.

To the adult reader, Kitty is obviously a young prostitute working the docks, but as a child I simply assumed she had run away because she was ashamed of something, perhaps lying or stealing. At the denouement, when Meg's father finally gets home, Kitty runs into Mrs Blossom from the bakery, who recognizes her as her lost daughter, 'Posy'. The two join Meg's family to sail to new beginnings abroad where even 'fallen women' can start afresh, perhaps in Australia like the Peggotys, the Micawbers and Em'ly's friend, Martha, at the end of Dickens' *David Copperfield*. Hesba Stretton's depiction of Kitty is sympathetic but unsentimental, and as a child I found the way Kitty helped Meg far more believable than the unmotivated interventions of wealthy Christian benefactors in some of the more formulaic of my grandmother's now forgotten prize novels. The example of Meg's heroic care for her siblings has remained a deep-buried template in my life (reinforced by other children's novels, such as *Little Women*), as it has for my daughter.

The Jessica novels

There is no obvious sexual theme in Hesba Stretton's Jessica novels, except perhaps in the unstated implication of Jessica's mother's life. But there is certainly a gender theme, though not quite as Callum Brown's analysis might predict. The salvation narrative in both books centres on the way Jessica's childish helplessness and trust acts as a catalyst for the moral awakening of the two men who befriend her, the elderly coffee stall owner who is also pew opener in the church where she creeps for refuge, and the minister of the church. The coffee seller/pew opener is saved from his avarice and the minister from pride in the charismatic preaching that attracts his large, fashionable congregation. Sexual temptation appears nowhere in the roster of their sins. Both men show generosity but also self-love and pride. Even Jessica's drunken mother is a mixture of angry possessiveness and pathos.

Her Benny

Silas Hocking's *Her Benny* also starts in a slum, this time in Liverpool, with two young siblings caring for each other. Their drunken father and cruel stepmother abuse and exploit them after their loving mother's death from what adults would have recognized as tuberculosis. In much the same way as in *Little Meg's Children*, the memory of their mother protects the children from temptation after they run away the first time their father beats Nelly. Their precarious independent life on the street, Nelly selling matches and Benny running errands and carrying bags, is eased by Joe, the nightwatchman, who is touched by Nelly's innocence and frailty, which he thinks marks her out from the other 'street Arabs'. Joe persuades a kindly widow to give them a place to sleep. When she reads Bible stories to Nelly, Benny is inspired to teach himself to read (much as 'Gypsy' Smith did in real life).[4] In the winter cold, Benny is providentially saved from the temptation to steal a woollen jacket for Nelly when she arrives unexpectedly early to meet him and touches his arm at the crucial moment. Hocking uses Perks, a hardened young thief, to voice the impossibility of living an honest life in such circumstances when the grown-up Benny takes 'the Word of God' to a Liverpool prison (Hocking nd, p 239). Perks plays the role of Tempter at dramatic junctures in the story but simultaneously is victim of harsh circumstance. Several 'angels in the house' in this early part of the story include the children's dead mother, Nelly herself and the kind widow.

The crux of the plot comes when Nelly is knocked over by a big dog. The fall compounds her 'wasting' state and she dies in hospital. On her deathbed, Nelly has a vision of heaven which I always found embarrassing and tended to skip over, though Benny's inconsolable grief at his sister's death I found devastating and entirely convincing. The only almost-direct allusion to the sexual moral of the evangelical narrative comes much later in the story when the adult Benny revisits Nelly's grave and wonders whether her early death perhaps saved her from some worse fate in the Liverpool slums, though there was so much that was terrible about that life of poverty and want that sexual shame never crossed my child's mind. I re-read the first part of the story many times as a child and found the second half, about Benny's growing up, much less involving. When I returned to the book after more than seventy years, I had forgotten most of what happened after Nelly's tragedy with the big black dog. What I had found so compelling were the struggles of slum children of my own age trying to survive and help each other with some sort of integrity.

The child Benny speaks a not always convincing working-class Liverpool patois and is perpetually cheerful, funny and hopeful like a boy in a cartoon or in a picaresque episode from Dickens, while Nelly has numerous fictional sisters, particularly Little Nell from Dickens' *Old Curiosity Shop*. The second half of the novel is much closer to the evangelical narrative of Callum Brown's model, being both the salvation story of Benny's self-formation and ultimately the romance of finding his ideal marriage partner, 'his own angel in the house' as Hocking actually puts it. The figure of the grown-up Benny has more than a touch of muscular Christianity and a good dose of the Protestant ethic. He resembles the youngest Cheeryble brother in Dickens' *Nicholas Nickleby*, cheerful, hard-working, loyal, grateful and unfailingly courteous, with the evangelical bonus of being educated through the Methodist chapel and evening classes, and proving heroic into the bargain.

Her Benny becomes the standard romance with a happy ending for the unflawed hero, who had tramped out of Liverpool after a mistaken accusation of theft but triumphs over misfortune and temptation through self-discipline, education, loyalty and hard work. He becomes an indispensable worker for the farming family that takes him in, he educates himself through the local Methodist church and is eventually reunited with his childhood heroine from Liverpool after saving her from a carriage accident. To the adult eye, the novel is too dependent on unlikely coincidence, with often unsubtle character description and an over-sharp division of good and bad, reward and punishment, especially by comparison with the potent ambiguities of Hesba Stretton's best novels – Hocking even has the repentant and despairing father of Benny and Nelly drown himself in the dock when he fails to find his misused children, in an obvious echo of Judas' suicide in the Christian Passion story.

Moral versus literary assessments of popularity: Arnold Bennett

Jan Susina reports that Hesba Stretton's style, if not her evangelical message, was admired by Thomas Hardy, who appreciated her unblinking depiction of life at the bottom of the social pile, as did Cardinal Newman, E.E. Nesbitt, Charlotte Yonge and other 'serious' writers (Susina 2009, chapter 8). Silas Hocking has not received, nor perhaps warranted, similar literary appreciation, although Philip Larkin noted laconically that as late as 1943, when he was first working as a librarian, the old folk of the North were still prepared to struggle up difficult dark staircases in wartime just to find Silas Hocking novels (Davenport 2015). Almost half a century before Larkin, Arnold Bennett published a book in which he uses Silas Hocking as the type case of the 'popular' as distinct from the 'artistic' fiction writer and does so with a sharp, satirical edge at Hocking's expense while marvelling at Hocking's unrivalled popular sales (Bennett 1901, pp 143–68). Bennett's book appeared while he was a full-time journalist, just before he gave up editing a pioneer woman's magazine (of which he was part owner) for the novels that by the time of the First World War had made him rich and famous. Bennett seems to have used this collection of his early reviews for

The Academy (Bennett's most recent biographer describes them as 'highbrow cultural columns on favourite authors') to work out the difference between 'artistic' and 'popular', perhaps in the hope of finding the secret of combining the two in high-quality fiction that was also lucrative.

At the time he wrote the original reviews, republished as *Faith and Fiction*, Bennett was working on his first novel, *The Man from the North* (published in 1898), written, as he later said, 'in the vein of the *écriture artiste*' (Carey 1992, p 154). The novel did not sell very well and made no money, though most critics regard it as a literary success. But Bennett learned from this first effort and perhaps from pondering what made for popular sales. Patrick Donovan, Bennett's latest biographer, in a chapter on Bennett's work in government propaganda under Max Beaverbrook during the First World War, comments on his 'preternatural ability to sense the tastes of the reading public' (Donovan 2022, p 141). His later novels were both critical and popular successes, bringing him both fame and fortune. The wide new readership made possible by mass schooling benefited Bennett just as surely as it provided the working-class readership of the prize books of Stretton and Hocking. John Carey begins his chapter on Bennett in *The Intellectuals and the Masses* with the large claim: 'Arnold Bennett is the hero of this book' (Carey 1992, p 152). Carey believes that among the novelists published between the late-19th and the mid-20th century Bennett uniquely narrowed the abyss between the masses and the intelligentsia, between popularity and artistic quality. The newly literate mass reading public of clerks and shopkeepers that emerged in the wake of the Education Act 1870 not only read his novels but saw their lives and concerns reflected in them. Bennett's leading protagonists are mostly members of the growing lower middle classes, out of which Bennett himself rose, although the lower classes of the Potteries also figure in his most admired works. These 'clerks' and 'shopkeepers' were scorned and patronized, as he was, by high-brow writers of the period, whose use of abstraction, erudite allusions and what he decried as the 'dandyism of technique' Bennett actively disliked and criticized ruthlessly in *Fame and Fiction* (Bennett 1901/2018, p 6).

Bennett's introductory chapter in *Fame and Fiction* presents it as a disinterested analysis of the qualities that distinguish 'popular' from 'artistic' fiction. In the review essays that follow, especially the one on Silas Hocking, examples of the disdain of the 'artist' for the 'popular' are hammered home. Yet Bennett is convinced that 'the average reader' respects and loves books that express 'some central righteousness ... at which it is impossible to sneer' and that 'average' readers of popular fiction can always detect calculating insincerity in an author. They expect grandeur of subject, imposing plots, heroic characters and fine actions although they neglect the architecture of the whole in favour of 'passing details and titillation' and demand happy endings rather than realism (Bennett 1901/2018, p 10).

In due course, Arnold Bennett became the scourge of cultural snobbery, particularly through a long-running feud with Virginia Woolf, who published a dismissive essay on his work in 1924 when she was a far less celebrated writer than the enormously popular Bennett. John Carey believes Woolf's disdain was misconceived, while Margaret Drabble, another of Bennett's biographers, believes that the root of their spat was class antagonism far more than disagreements over 'realist' as against 'Modernist' style, or over 'feminism' or literary quality (Carey 1992, pp 152–81; see also Drabble 1986, 2022).

Bennett begins his chapter on Silas Hocking in *Fame and Fiction* by puzzling over 'the dazzling and marvellous secret' of 'probably the most popular of living novelists' (with almost two million sales the previous year) (Bennett 1901, p 145). Bennett asks rhetorically; Why can Hocking's novels not be found in Westminster bookshops when they sell hugely in Cornwall and the industrial towns of the Midlands and the North? Answer: because 'his fame is rooted in Dissent' and 'Kensington never dissents'. His books are stocked in abundance by bookshops in the Midlands and northern English provincial towns, the home of Dissent. Hocking's fiction is everything Bennett deplores about the Dissent that so oppressed his own childhood as eldest son and heir of a controlling, ambitious, self-educated solicitor. Bennett's father began as a draper and pawnbroker and he forced his family to attend the Primitive Methodist chapel in Burslem while staying at home himself. Donovan (2022, p 23) quotes Arnold as saying: 'I preferred damnation to conversion, it is less humiliating.' In the essay on Hocking, Bennett (1901/2018, p 147) deplores the Dissenting didacticism, moralism, suspicion of the arts, 'apart from hymns and *The Messiah*', of Hocking's style and its demand that 'print literature must behave itself'. Restraint is Hocking's watchword, sensational stuff occurs offstage or is over swiftly. Above all, Hocking rejects realism and displays 'conspicuous avoidance of the intellect' which, Bennett presumes, is reserved for theology, politics and business. Hocking's books offer only 'tepid scenes of sentiment' because his 'tact' and 'reticence' 'must respectfully kneel to the current religious and spiritual ideal' and not 'incommode the most tender susceptibility' (Bennett 1901/2018, pp 147–148, 150–151). Bennett examines one of Hocking's novels, *The Day of Recompense*, to show how it exemplifies the literary faults of popular fiction – improbable coincidences, melodramatic plots, 'all the play of character is tremendously simplified', 'every complication beyond the main one is neatly nipped in the bud' (Bennett 1901/2018, p 151). Bennett's case for the prosecution ends with a rhetorical flourish explaining why such technically inferior stuff is so popular: its author 'is the Methodist million made vocal' (Bennett 1901/2018, pp 148–51). Bennett, the defiant unbeliever, is repelled, as secularists like Callum Brown are, by the 'simplistic' moral messages of the evangelical narrative, but even more by its failures of taste and style. Arnold Bennett's own fictions are emphatically not examples of the evangelical narrative and, for him, Silas Hocking's worst offence is the literary equivalent of the quip Noel Coward gives Amanda in *Private Lives*: 'strange how potent cheap music is'. Bennett ends his chapter on Hocking by throwing up his hands:

> What is that quality lurking in every sentence, on every page, which attracts? To this question, though I have approached it sympathetically and without arrogance, I find no answer. When souls call aloud to each other in the night, each knows its fellow: and that is all one can say. (Bennett 1901, p 153)

Identity, gender and class: the end of the feminization of piety?

As a child just beginning to read real books, I found the stories by Hesba Stretton and Silas Hocking far more compelling than anything I was given at primary school. I found Peter Pan's struggles with Captain Hook alarmingly exciting when the book was read aloud to us in primary school, but I didn't recognize or identify at all with the (middle-class) Darling family, not even with limply nurturing Wendy. Yet the stories of Little Meg and Benny were almost equally powerful pictures of poor but valiant slum children that I immediately recognized as earlier versions of 'my tribe', in the way the Edwardian lower middle classes had seen their own tribe in the fictions of Arnold Bennett. The conditions my grandparents had lived in were not so different from those of Meg and Benny. The poor and outcast, especially children, were the central characters in these stories: their actions, choices and struggles for dignity *mattered*; they were heroic. The prize novels were my earliest spur to political and social awareness. Their moral lessons did not seem essentially gendered: Benny cared for his sister and Meg cared for her brother and the baby. I never recognized the 'angels in the house' as having much to do with the real women who cared for me, and I never intuited any message about sexual morality. The message I heard was Christian love for family and neighbour, however poor or young you might be, the importance of honesty and generosity, and the repeated warning never to mistake respectability for Christian virtue or for 'importance'.

Popular 'evangelical' fiction of this kind was undoubtedly consequential in planting the moral priority of caring for others in generations of working-class women, often as part of a moral hope of better things which expected more of men, not least that they should be responsible and loving husbands and fathers.[5] This is clearly part of what Mary Harrington refers to as the 'rules' that hedged around sex before it was loosed into modern 'liberation'. I find it easy to understand why the (now-secular) popular family sagas like the ones my mother read in her old age and TV soap operas today are read and watched avidly by (older) working-class women precisely because they continue the theme of women's pivotal importance to the continuity and solidarity of families and communities, especially in bad times. It seems to me much more doubtful that the popular evangelical narrative was *as* powerful in passing on the double standard of sexual morality. That, as all the research shows, was largely sustained through the sexual culture and actual behaviour of the peer group and was enforced by community sanctions for breaches of 'respectability' – and it dispensed with direct religious justification quite readily. The social and material cost of unmarried motherhood, in particular, was always heavy, and it was women who paid it. The connection between sexual mores and respectability was patchily maintained until women got more or less effective control of their own fertility and, for some of them, the ability to earn decent incomes for themselves. There was an awkward transition from at least the Second World War to the early 1990s when, for young women, the consequences of sex before or outside marriage remained not much more predictable than playing Russian roulette. Even in an era of supposedly emancipated sexuality, the sexual bargain, especially its power imbalance, is in practice still largely tilted toward the male, as Joan Wallach Scott, Louise Perry and Mary Harrington insist.

Does anything still remain of the feminization of piety? Even if women in general are no longer 'the pious sex', in the shrunken congregations of the Christian churches women are still in the majority and they constitute an increasing proportion of leaders, priests and ministers (not least because secularization has made it a less status-bearing occupation for men) even though the very top still tends to remain out of women's reach. Perhaps the most long-lasting legacy of the feminization of piety is the still powerful assumption that females are responsible for the bulk of the caring work that energizes community and bonds and anchors the family, whether there is an effective father in it or not, and irrespective of whether it is a hybrid mix of parentage. It does not even depend on a conversion experience like Mary Harrington's to reclaim the virtue and satisfactions of 'care' in motherhood. An episode of the Radio 4 series, *Life Changing*, in 2021, told the story of a young woman, home schooled and brought up by her mother in the counterculture, who at the end of her university degree did not think twice about adopting her two young half-siblings after her mother died in Spain and her alcoholic step-father lost his children to Spanish social services (Garvey and Beere 2022). She may never have read Hesba Stretton but, like many other women, she had undoubtedly absorbed by an invisible osmosis, perhaps from her own mother and the surrounding 'secular' culture, the injunction to care for her siblings, at whatever cost to her own immediate desires. However far the sexual and gender bargain may have shifted, women remain the caring sex and the backbone of the 'caring sector' of the economy.

Residues of the evangelical narrative in contemporary secular culture: social protest and the church as villain

Since the high noon of the evangelical narrative, popular fiction, plays, films, television documentaries and other imaginative forms have continued to carry social reform messages, but in increasingly secularized packages. That message is still urgent. Old and new forms of popular culture plead the case of care for the poor and marginalized in exposures of the failings and gaps in the welfare state, the increasing inequalities in the workings of 'late' capitalism and the patterns of exploitation that shift from one to the next sector of social and economic life. The 2020 Booker Prize winner, *Shuggy Bain*, is a fictionalized memoir of the author's alcoholic mother, abandoned with her three children by her philandering second husband, and the struggles of the family when they are rehoused in a tough mining community (Stuart 2020). In common with the genre of 'misery memoirs', such novels are anatomies of social problems but seldom blueprints for reform.

Not only print fiction but television, streaming services and other digital outlets distribute socially engaged works such as Ken Loach's films which in a speech at St Martin in the Fields in 2023 he described as 'films that give voice to the voiceless'. They castigate the failings of the benefits system, *I, Daniel Blake*, of the precarious and exploitative 'gig economy', *Sorry We Missed You*, and racism in the film about Syrian refugees in a small village near Durham, *The Old Oak*. Small Axe, a series of films by Steve McQueen shown on the BBC in 2021, also expose British racism. They continue Hesba Stretton's and Silas Hocking's themes of chronic social problems that urgently need to be addressed, but the narrative is now shorn of its evangelical frame and often placed in a more explicitly political one instead. Care for others, especially the needs of the poor and marginalized, is still the point of the message but mostly divorced from the original Christian rationale, which has been thoroughly 'occluded' when not roundly repudiated. A good example of this is the television film *Help!* (subtitled *No One is Coming*), written by Jack Thorne and directed by Marc Munden, first screened on Channel 4 in September 2021. It portrays an untrained young carer, played by a popular actress, Jodie Comer, starting work in a residential care home at the height of the COVID-19 pandemic and finding it (realistically) drastically understaffed and grossly short of personal protective equipment and other resources. The film follows her struggle to provide effective care in these circumstances, focusing on one middle-aged resident with early-onset dementia to highlight the management's dubious recourse to heavy sedation as the only way to contain problems. Even when the Labour Party's fortunes are at a low ebb, the reform message and the moral outrage in productions like this are likely to be understood as a legacy of the British political Left, without recognizing the considerable debt of the Left to its Dissenting forebears. The churches are usually absent from these popular tales or, sometimes with good cause, cast as villains, as, for instance, in the 2013 film *Philomena*, adapted from the book by journalist Martin Sixsmith which exposes historical abuses in mother and baby homes for unmarried women in Ireland and is regularly screened on terrestrial television (Sixsmith 2009).

Although ever-increasing numbers of people simply discarded substantive belief, many of them, like Deborah Orr's parents, kept or even strengthened their hold on the rules of respectability, especially over family and sexual morality, and still associated it with the churches they no longer attended and the Bible they no longer read. This was particularly true for the older generations during the transition period between the 1950s and the 1990s, when changes in the gender order were being accepted among younger generations, though in a staggered and far from uniform fashion. Nothing illustrates this more clearly than the protests, receiving escalating publicity in the last decade, by women who were effectively coerced into handing over their babies for adoption by 'moral pressure' from their families, doctors and nurses, the churches and some of the church-run mother and baby homes to which they were sent when they were pregnant but unmarried between the 1950s and the late 1970s. Television programmes such as the ITV series *Long Lost Family* serve to keep this issue fresh in the public mind. This practice was by no means universal and in some places families, with various degrees of reluctance, accepted the child, or the father might have been living in an informal household with the mother, or the mother might even have been able to afford to keep the child, particularly once the state provided an income through welfare benefits. Yet it is striking that in the postwar period up to the 1960s, 40 per cent of illegitimate children were legally adopted by one or both of their birth parents. Elizabeth Roberts' oral history of the Manchester area also makes clear that up to the 1950s many people were less disapproving of a woman who kept her child than of one who let it go for adoption outside the extended family (Roberts 1995). Even so, around 250,000 illegitimate babies born in Britain between the end of the Second World War and the 1970s were taken from their often very young mothers by what many now describe as 'forced adoption'. A petition from around 300 of these women was given to the Prime Minister in May 2021 calling for an official apology from Parliament; the Movement for an Adoption Apology, after several years of activity, collected signatures online to support the petition. Some of the women described the brutal removal of their babies as 'kidnapping' and many suffered long-lasting trauma from the experience, describing punitive attitudes in NHS maternity hospitals, where some of the women were denied pain relief in labour because they had been 'bad' and needed to remember the pain. Perhaps this rationale rested, though probably at some removes, on a hyper-literal reading of the Genesis creation myth in which the pain of childbirth is part of God's punishment after the Fall (men were doomed to work 'by the sweat of [their] brow' in order to eat). The Scottish, the Welsh and the Westminster parliaments conducted investigations of forced adoptions between 2022 and 2023, and the Scottish and Welsh governments have issued formal apologies while Westminster has expressed 'regrets'.

The National Council for the Unmarried Mother and Her Child, now Gingerbread, worked to make it possible for unmarried mothers to keep their children and had some success in changing attitudes in Church of England moral welfare homes and more generally after the Second World War. Adoption was regularized and 'professionalized' by the Children Act 1975 and the Adoption Act 1976. Until the latter Act implemented the recommendations of the 1972 Houghton Committee report, adoption had often been a haphazard and private process without any systematic checks on either private arrangements or the policies of adoption agencies, which were often run by churches. The whole history of unmarried motherhood is lucidly analysed by Pat Thane and Tanya Evans, showing the vicissitudes in policy and practice in this area from the First World War to the present day (Thane and Evans 2012).

Christian care for neighbour versus respectability and institutional interest

The example of forced adoption illustrates the divided priorities of the churches. The tension between the traditional role of the churches policing the boundary of morality and respectability and their mission to give care to those who need it is responsible for the churches now being cast as hypocrites and villains in some contemporary cultural expressions of indignation about chronic social problems and injustices. Care for others is widely accepted as the distinctive mark of Christians, yet the churches have so publicly torn themselves apart over changes in gender roles and sexual mores since the second half of the 20th century, that that struggle has often swamped the care imperative. Sexuality and sexual morality have sometimes seemed to be the only kind of sin (or flouting of respectability) serious enough to divide Christian from Christian and from fellow citizens. Jessica Martin, my daughter, argues that this foregrounding of sexuality in the moral priorities and internal war of the institutional churches may well be the unconscious import of contemporary secular culture's overvaluation of sex. She writes, as an Anglican priest and theologian: 'Suppose that our division was itself handed to the Church on the back of a general cultural idolization of sex as transcendent liberation, and that the Church has ever since been breaking itself to pieces on a rock carved with the features of a secular idol?' (Martin 2020, p 101).

That internal struggle in the churches over sexuality still dominates the news about religious matters in the secular press and can hardly fail to leave its mark on secular assumptions about Christians that cast a shadow on the notion of Christians as 'caring'. The formal opposition of the Roman Catholic and Anglican Churches to same-sex unions when they were made legal in British law in 2014 was all but incomprehensible to the secular population of the country, particularly among younger generations. The more recent decision of the Synod of the Church of England to countenance limited prayers of blessing but not the marriage of same-sex partners has done little to change that or to reassure the liberal members of the Church who continue to hope for full rights for LGBTQ+ Christians in the Church of England in line with changes in some other denominations.

Public awareness of the negative side of the churches' image has been compounded by the very long resistance in the Roman Catholic and Anglican Churches to recognizing and confronting a persistent pattern of sexual abuse of children, young people and vulnerable adults by a minority of clergy. Church hierarchies have consistently protected the reputation of the institution rather than the victims of the abuse. There have been attempts, mainly from victims and their champions, to bring the issue to light since at least the 1970s but without results for over forty years. Both Ireland and Britain finally launched national independent inquiries on the issue. Ireland saw a sequence of inquiries between 2005 and 2021 dealing with different Roman Catholic dioceses and both clerical sexual abuse and the abusive practices towards unmarried mothers in mother and baby homes. In Britain the Anglican and Roman Catholic Churches saw independent inquiries into the sexual abuse of children and vulnerable adults, published in 2019 and 2020, respectively (Independent Inquiry into Child Sexual Abuse 2019; Independent Inquiry into Child Sexual Abuse 2020). Both Churches have acknowledged their failures and set in train new systems of safeguarding, but the culture around sexuality is deep-rooted and not easy to shift. Pope Francis had the Code of Canon Law changed in 2021 to categorize sexual abuse as a crime against human dignity rather than against chastity. The Anglican Independent Inquiry into Child Sexual Abuse in 2019 reported that there was a culture of secrecy around sexuality and an unwillingness to examine the issue; a minority who conflated homosexuality with child abuse; an anti-women sentiment among some Anglican clergy; a deferential culture that protected clergy who were accorded 'privilege, respect and reverence'; and a tendency for clergy to close ranks to protect their 'tribe'. The Executive Summary of the Inquiry concluded that 'the culture of the Church of England facilitated it becoming a place where abusers could hide' (Independent Inquiry into Child Sexual Abuse 2019). The efforts of senior clerics to find ways of forgiving the abusers, often moving them to new parishes where many of them continued to abuse, was strongly criticized, and new safeguarding arrangements took the executive function in child abuse cases out of episcopal hands and invested it in an independent office. The issue rumbles on even under new safeguarding arrangements, which are often box-ticking exercises rather than attempts to tackle deep-seated cultural attitudes in the institutional churches. Fictionalized treatments of clerical abuse have featured in popular television dramas and novels such as Sebastian Barry's powerful *Old God's Time*, which pivots around the Irish scandal (Barry 2023).

Identical problems and responses have been found in other Western societies. Robert Orsi, one of the primary researchers in a large research programme based in the University of Notre Dame, Indiana, on child abuse in the American Roman Catholic Church, has interviewed survivors and, like the Independent Inquiry in the Church of England, he finds the sacred authority of clergy acts as a facilitator of abuse and a cause of the displaced guilt and long-term mental ill health of many victims.[6]

The Reverend Richard Coles, an Anglican parish priest who is also a writer and well-known broadcaster spent the decade or so after graduating in the 1980s as keyboard player for indie band *The Communards*, and he was a member of the political initiative Red Wedge, living a life of protest, gay sex, party drugs and rock 'n' roll. When its joys soured, he converted to Roman Catholicism and briefly considered a monastic vocation. In his memoir of the period, *Fathomless Riches: Or How I Went from Pop to Pulpit*, he recounts one of the signposts on his route 'home' to Anglicanism when he made his confession in Rome to an American Franciscan priest and encountered an unbridgeable difference of convictions. He writes:

> When I seek the Church's forgiveness and counsel in matters of sexuality it is not because I think it is in itself wrong. I think it is the morally neutral context in which my less than loving, less than generous actions occur – that's where the trouble lies – and no matter how much the Church may want me to, I cannot repent of a sin that I do not think a sin. … However, I needed the Church to be more attentive, more forbearing, more clear-sighted, more just, more loving, in my relationships with other people, the person with whom I was only glancingly involved, and especially those with whom I would much rather not be involved at all. (Coles 2015, p 234)

This, in a nutshell, delineates the area in which the respectability/sexual morality border patrols of the churches tend to run up against differently calibrated ethical and religious judgements about the nature of sexual sin, wherever the erotic activity and feeling lies in the range of sexual orientation. It reinforces the argument that sexual issues may have been given a disproportionate dominance in the roster of human evil whether the prevailing sexual mores have been restrictive or permissive – after all, it is the temptations of power not of sex that figure in the Gospel accounts of Jesus' temptations on the wilderness. It is quite true that sexual life provides ample occasions for unkindness, exploitation, cruelty, betrayal, selfishness and violence, usually involving the misuse of power, but that does not intrinsically distinguish it from other arenas such as economic and political life. That was Richard Coles' point. After his male partner, who was also an Anglican priest, died in 2019, Cole received abusive letters from fellow clerics convinced homosexuality was absolutely wrong, some of them rejoicing that he and his much-loved partner would both fry in hell for eternity (see Coles 2021). Here, the value of caring is trumped by an inflexible rule which encapsulates the letter writers' punitive version of Christian sexual codes. Coles and his partner had been required by the Church to take a vow of celibacy in order to live together in one vicarage, and they were forbidden to offer 'blessings' in church to other same-sex couples. Coles was a notably successful parish priest but retired early in 2022, retreating into writing and broadcasting, 'tired of being a warrior' after a dispiriting, exhausting and frustrating decade on the Church barricades defending the dignity and rights of LGBTQ+ Christians, many of whom, as he says, are in same-sex relationships 'full of grace and truth' that the Church should be celebrating (Coles, quoted in Moran 2022).

Younger generations in the British population have very little time for such sexual taboos and are ruthless in condemning hypocrisy in the institutional churches. As we saw in Chapter 3, research on Gen Z by Katz and colleagues shows widespread acceptance of fluid sexualities and readiness to pursue sex for recreational and strictly uncommitted pleasure with multiple partners, largely using online dating, during a period now often seen as an extended adolescent stage of life (Katz et al 2021). They try to keep emotion and commitments out of the picture. They mistrust the authoritarian, hierarchical, patriarchal nature of formal institutions and the few religious members in the Gen Z sample reject any rules and dogmas of their churches that contradict their own values of individual autonomy, authenticity, diversity, tolerance and acceptance of others. In spite of the dubious and potentially toxic aspects of the culture of 'sexual freedom' in the West, among this generation it is still important to care for others, including protecting the right of all individuals to judge for themselves on all matters that are important to them. We have seen that many of them weigh care for self and for others equally and that we do not yet know what form their families will take, how stable their eventual commitments, if any, will prove to be or whether the burden of everyday care will still fall disproportionately on women. At all events, the sexual component in the evangelical narrative of Callum Brown's thesis seems to be nowhere in the lives of Gen Z. Perhaps, rather than warring over what is and is not 'marriage', and what precisely counts as sexual 'sin', the churches might more persuasively urge the rewards of commitment and support consideration for the needs of others, not just in sexual relationships but in life more widely, including in the many blended or reconstituted families and both heterosexual and same-sex households struggling to create stability and a nurturing domestic life, who sometimes look for support and acceptance from their local priest and parish community.

Performance poetry and moral indignation

And what of social outrage? In the old industrial cities where ethnic minorities and the poor, today's equivalent of Meg and Benny, still cluster, contemporary performance poetry is a genre that has a considerable presence and often takes for its themes the same indignation about marginalization and exclusion that fired Hesba Stretton and Silas Hocking. But it tends to see religion as part of the problem rather than any part of the solution. Two powerful voices from the Manchester scene are Tony Walsh and Lemn Sissay, both writers and well-known performers. Walsh's double-punning performance name is 'Longfella' (a poet who is six and a half feet tall), and he puts into his poetry the experience of years in and around Manchester as a social worker who knows local working-class people intimately. He wrote and performed a poem in memory of the victims of the terrorist bombing at the Ariana Grande concert at the Manchester Arena in 2017. The BBC has given him a platform, as have several arts festivals, including Glastonbury. Sissay is an award-winning poet, writer and broadcaster who appears frequently on the BBC and at arts festivals. He has received awards and honours from several universities, including a decade as Chancellor of Manchester University, and he has been a Booker Prize judge and was the official poet to the 2012 Olympics. He received an MBE in 2010 and an OBE in 2021. He supports education for Black males and anti-racist initiatives, and he quietly concerns himself with 'looked-after' children, or children in care. His bestselling memoir, *My Name is Why*, and a number of related film documentaries give an account of his childhood in Wigan as the illegitimate child of a young Ethiopian visiting student who left him in Britain after birth (Sissay 2019). From babyhood, he was fostered by a strict Baptist family who originally intended to adopt him but handed him back to the local authority at the age of 12. After the sudden repudiation by the only family he had ever known and bleak, often racist experiences in a series of children's homes and schools, he found his voice and eventually became part of the Manchester performance scene, to which he gravitated soon after he left care.

Themes that feature often in Sissay's poetry, especially his early work, are the damage inflicted by racism and by children's homes that are so impersonally controlling that they can be experienced as 'home' by nobody: care is nowhere to be found. One striking poem, 'Fallen', however, is a tender defence of young single mothers like his own, caught on the cusp between child and woman; it is an understated protest at the tyranny of respectability and religious condemnation that lay behind his mother's leaving him behind in England when she went home to her Pentecostal family in Ethiopia after his birth (Sissay 2017, p 196). One of his aubades, the untitled quatrains he has written every day on waking for the past ten years, is full of painful longing for his mother (Sissay 2023, p 92). Another is a wry comment on the unwelcoming, ungenerous English and the strident certainty of churches expressed in the deceptively simple verse form of a nursery rhyme (Sissay 2023, p 141). His choice of adjectives such as 'little' (repeated), 'pointy', 'angry', 'shouty' makes it a vivid evocation of hectoring small-mindedness.

Much of Tony Walsh's poetry is about the lives of the marginalized lowest class of the North West, the unemployed and underemployed men and women on 'zero hours' and other 'shit work' in the 'precariat', the women still trying to take care of their kids against all odds, often alone and with too little money coming in, consoling themselves as and when they can with fags and booze, sex and rock 'n' roll, but sometimes, more hopefully, in libraries with books. His tone is sympathetic and comprehending, and his Lancashire women are wholly familiar to me. They are not 'angels in the house' but they care for their kids and for others as best they can. One poignant poem, 'Mother's Day', with audible echoes of Hesba Stretton, is about the anguish, anger and regret that surges through a men's prison on that peak day for suicides (Walsh 2013, pp 94–5). Tony Walsh addresses the angry and despised who have 'tiny dreams' of dignity and respect: the overwhelmed young mother who found a fleeting semblance of love before he left; the 'bastard' condemned as 'nothing' by 'the pastors and her masters' (Walsh 2013, p 56). In this poem, 'Tiny Dreams', Walsh urges these women to try the magic of words, bringing all the frustrations, the violence and despair, the pleasures, tasteful and tawdry, the full experience of being alive, to the poetry everyone has it in them to write.

Tony Walsh sings and snarls about domestic violence, lack of work and lack of money, quiet or violent despair, and he celebrates the ordinary and extraordinary pleasures of love, music and words. His poetry is not at all religious and some of his oppressors are 'the pastors and masters' of 'Tiny Dreams', while many of his villains have lives as hopeless as those of the victims. The route out of degradation is not evangelical conversion but finding your own voice to tell your own story to the people in your community. His audience may be smaller than Hesba Stretton's but Walsh's social indignation is in direct genealogical line from the 'street Arab' novels, and his message is continuous with the Christian vision of transforming the world to eliminate injustice just as we also see in the secularized indignation of feminism and the civil rights movements.

6

Feminism and the Gendering of Care

Drudgery

I begin by exploring the 'drudgery' of domestic labour and caring, starting from its place in Christian values. George Herbert's poem 'The Elixir' has been familiar to churchgoers for many generations as a hymn: 'Teach me my God and king', number 790 in *Hymns Ancient and Modern*. It expresses the Christian value of seeing God in all things and doing even the most menial work on behalf of others as if for God Himself, which, in the phrase from verse 5, 'makes drudgery divine' (Herbert 1633/2017, p 291). It mirrors Jesus' own understanding of his calling as the 'Servant King', the divine ruler who is 'servant' or 'slave' of others, which he dramatized by doing the customary work of a slave when he washed his disciples' feet at the beginning of the Passion narrative. This symbolic representation of the Christian moral inversion of hierarchy and power relations is liturgically re-enacted on Maundy Thursday in the ceremony of foot washing. The moral and spiritual value of menial work done for others has been obscured, maybe even lost, over the course of my lifetime. Yet no comparable secular validation of drudgery as a positive virtue has replaced it. Moreover, despite the Reverend George Herbert's justly celebrated saintliness, as a well-born 17th-century gentleman, he would never literally have 'swept a room' in his rectory, as he recommended in the poem. That kind of domestic labour, however symbolically Christ-like, was the proper province of women and servants. If drudgery were not the common lot of people of little or no importance, the moral inversion of its status would lack symbolic power.

Christian artists of many kinds have found inspiration in that transformative image. The painter Stanley Spencer was introduced to the *Confessions* of St Augustine by a fellow artist from the Slade while he was working as the lowliest of orderlies for up to 15 hours a day at Beaufort military hospital in the early part of the First World War, before he was sent to the front in Macedonia. Augustine's depiction of the nature of God transformed Spencer's understanding of his back-breaking menial labour into a belief that he was cooperating in God's continuous creative work in the world – 'ever busy yet ever at rest', in Augustine's words. In her chapter on Spencer's art, Frances Spalding highlights his inclusion of drudges like himself, the baggage handlers, cleaners and stretcher bearers, as crucial figures in the visionary murals in Sandham Memorial Chapel at Burghclere, in which he depicts the resurrection of soldiers from both sides killed on the Macedonian battlefield and their handing in their crosses to Christ (Spalding 2022, pp 169–85). Spalding quotes Spencer's remark to a friend that when he arrives at the entrance to heaven, he will tell God to 'take into consideration the number of men I have cleaned and the amount of *floors* I have *scrubbed*, as well as the excellence of my pictures so as to let me in' (Spalding 2022, p 176).

As we have seen in earlier chapters, some Christian women, including the Victorian poet Elizabeth Barrett Browning, as well as many secular ones have nevertheless deplored women's routine domestic drudgery and caring duties as hindrances to any artistic achievement or socially valued work they might otherwise do.[1] In 1895, at the age of 19, Gwen John left the family home in Tenby to study at the Slade alongside her younger brother, Augustus. From this time on, she lived in sparsely furnished rented rooms, first in London and after 1904 in Paris, until the later years in Meudon when she finally acquired her own house. She financed her painting for many years by working as an artist's model and openly took, probably two, male lovers, the most important being the French sculptor Rodin, for whom she modelled and with whom she studied; there may also have been affairs with women after the Rodin period. Gwen John became a passionate but not always conforming Roman Catholic in her maturity after Rodin ended the affair, which had lasted around a decade, but she never endorsed the Victorian and Edwardian model of the 'good woman'. Early in her career as an artist she wrote a note to remind herself that her life could itself be a work of art and a beacon of hope to others, but that she should not waste it 'thinking of little ways of helping people', as women in her time were expected to do (Foster 2023, p 20).

Women writers, musicians and artists have alternative Christian resources in the Gospels, for instance, in the parable of the talents or Jesus' injunction not to hide your light under a bushel, which can be read as instruction to use God-given abilities. Yet some women artists and writers have willingly accepted tasks that Elizabeth Barrett Browning and Gwen John regarded as pure burden and waste, and some have even embraced them as intrinsic parts of their creative work. Among these is the Victorian Christian poet Christina Rossetti, a contemporary of Barrett Browning. Christina Rossetti is as celebrated for her hymns as George Herbert for his – especially her Christmas carol 'In the bleak midwinter'. The Rossetti scholar Dinah Roe argues that Rossetti's 'reading diary', *Time Flies*, shows her creative response to the 'interruptions' to her thinking and writing that arose from having to care for her ailing and needy mother, two aunts and her frequently sick brother, Dante Gabriel, all of whom she shared a home with at some time (Roe 2022). Roe comments that caring is a persistent theme in Rossetti's poetry. It is not usually emphasized, but it leaped out at Roe during the pandemic lockdown in 2021 when she was working on a study of Rossetti's poetry while teaching university courses online from home at the same time as caring for, and home-schooling, her six-year-old child. Rossetti, like many other women of her period (and like many employed women confined to home in the COVID-19 pandemic), could only write (or 'work') in brief moments 'stolen' from urgent domestic and family duties. Roe sees evidence in Rossetti's texts that fragmentation and broken concentration are deployed within the form of the poetry itself, making a 'salvation' of it, both in a literary sense and by being 'an act of creative self-maintenance' on the part of the poet. In the diary, Rossetti describes these domestic 'interruptions' as 'Providential' and 'profitable' rather than 'vexatious', because they are 'sent us ... from without'. They were the spur that drove her to turn divided attention to spiritual and creative account (Roe 2022, p 13).[2]

The painter, sculptor and writer Maeve Gilmore was over a generation younger than Gwen John and Stanley Spencer, who were already working artists when she was born in 1917. Gilmore studied at the Westminster School of Art, where she met her husband, the artist and novelist Mervyn Peake, who taught there in the 1920s and 1930s. Gilmore was brought up in the Catholic Church but her art was not explicitly Christian, as Stanley Spencer's often was, even when his subjects were relocated to his native Cookham.[3] Gilmore drew her subjects largely from her own domestic life without explicit religious allusions, although it is clear that she retained a religious faith for much of her life.[4] With other members of the Peake family, her granddaughter, Christian Peake, set up an exhibition at Studio Voltaire of some twenty of the pictures left to her by Maeve Gilmore, on the one hundred and fifth anniversary of Gilmore's birth, hoping to alert a contemporary generation to the work of this virtually forgotten woman artist (Barnett and Peake 2022; Gilmore Archive 2022). The exhibition gathered appreciative notices. In one review, Francesca Wade notes that Gilmore always gave priority to her husband's work, especially after he developed Parkinson's disease (Wade 2022). She put caring for him and supporting his work as well as caring for their children ahead of her own art, as her memoir amply documents (Gilmore 1970). Gilmore decorated the interior walls of many of the rooms in her last house with murals, much as Vanessa Bell had done in Charleston.[5] She made an artistic virtue of her domestic constraints, remarking in her memoir, *A World Away*, that she was always able to concentrate intensely on a painting or an idea for one, even in the midst of the hurly burly of family life with three squabbling children, a sick husband and a need to support her husband's work – she was largely responsible for editing the last volume of his *Gormenghast* trilogy as his illness progressed (Gilmore 1970, p 110). She chose the subjects of her paintings from her own domestic life and that of other women, just as women artists like Mary Cassatt and Berthe Morisot had done. In her memoir, Gilmore comments: 'I painted a great deal from my children – using their play and their turmoil, boys on stilts, handstands, somersaulting, dressed up in Indian war-dress, trying to achieve the rhythm of their movements in simplified form' (Gilmore 1970, p 110). In Gilmore's modernist use of 'homely' subjects, Francesca Wade detects subtle allusions to other artists, including Piero della Francesca and the surrealist Dorothea Tanning. In her 'Woman's Hour' interview, Christian Peake remarks that although 'the domestic gaze' was not valued in her grandmother's time, today its artistic validity is better recognized (Barnett and Peake 2022). Francesca Wade draws particular attention to *Woman in Doorway*, a painting with Gilmore's signature positioned on the threshold between two rooms, in one of which a woman, Gilmore herself, bare to the waist, being her own artist's model, stands in shadow with raised arms, while in the other sunlight shines on a saucepan hanging on the wall. Wade points to the uncertainty here about whether home is 'the painter's prison or simply the frame that sets off her painting' (Wade 2022, p 32). An editorial on the exhibition in *The Guardian* selects another painting, 'Mother and Child', as the focus of a similar ambiguity – a naked toddler importunately tugs on his mother's dressing gown, uncovering her breasts, while the rose in his mother's hand, pointing towards the open space of the garden, casts a sinister shadow in the shape of a gun (The Guardian 2022). Christian Peake recalled her grandmother's eloquence about the toughness and restrictions of motherhood as well as its joys. Gilmore admits that she found it harder to be single-minded about her work later in life when the distractions of family life had fallen away, leaving her 'with more time and less friction', but it is likely that this was partly the effect of her acute and long-lasting sense of loss after the early death of her husband, her artistic partner and most constructive critic (Gilmore 1970, p 110).

A recent book by Jude Piesse, *The Ghost in the Garden: In Search of Darwin's Lost Garden*, shows a contemporary woman literary scholar making similar creative use of the constrained time when she was primary carer for her two very young daughters (Piesse 2021). Childcare inevitably ate away the time available for research and teaching, but she took the children on rambles through what remained of the garden of The Mount, the house in Shrewsbury where Charles Darwin grew up. This set her pondering the contribution to Darwin's early botanical investigations that came from his mother, a talented gardener and breeder of doves, as well as from his older sisters as they all worked, unremarked, as females did in all such middle-class households and gardens. Piesse then extended her initially desultory probing to following clues in the Darwin diaries, letters and other sources that suggest unacknowledged contributions by the female Darwins and by their labouring gardeners to the observations and experiments on plants and bees that Darwin made in his boyhood and young manhood at The Mount.

These are random instances of creative use being made of unavoidable 'drudgery' that happened to come to my notice as I planned this chapter, and a systematic search would doubtless throw up many more. They are the modern, real-life opposites of Mrs Jellyby in Dickens' satirical portrait of a woman who spends the time she 'ought' to devote to caring for her family and controlling her servants to raising funds for the African mission field instead. *Bleak House* is perhaps the most complete version of Callum Brown's 'evangelical narrative' among all Dickens' novels (Brown 2001), and his comic caricature of the 'unwomanly' Mrs Jellyby in that novel is today seen as misogynist, a charge now often levelled at his treatment of the real women in his life (Carey 1997; Tomalin 2012).[6] The ideal that Mrs Jellyby violates is the Victorian ideal of feminine domestic virtue. It has nothing to do with sexual purity but is all about women as carers. Unlike Mrs Jellyby, the women in my examples in this chapter willingly accept that duty of care in the family, and simply tuck in creative activity around it or even use it to stimulate the creative process. My examples all come from the arts and literary scholarship, where individual rather than collective work is a recognized option, and it might be harder to find examples among women doctors, business leaders, physical scientists or engineers, whose work is less easily conducted away from their professional laboratories, observatories, operating theatres and collaborative teams, even in our digitally connected age. Manifestly, the examples I cite do not turn all drudgery into a creative resource, or all drudges into artists: they are achievements 'against the odds', in defiance of the time and effort and the conventional negative value assigned to the whole range of necessary menial labour and caring. In the case of Jude Piesse, what stimulated her to write *The Ghost in the Garden* was precisely her consciousness of that conventional valuation, and what it conceals.

Feminist biographies of women, particularly of able women married to celebrated creative men, often highlight the way some wives, such as Eileen O'Shaughnessy, wife of George Orwell, sacrifice their own ambitions to support and sometimes to contribute directly to their husbands' work without ever being publicly acknowledged as co-creators, as well as taking on all the household drudgery and childcare (Oakley 2021; Topp 2021; Funder 2023). These are stories of the women who succumb, willingly or not, to the odds that are stacked against women's creativity in a 'man's world'.

Though lying beyond the direct cultural influence of the Christian ideas that informed Rossetti, Barrett Browning and Stanley Spencer, in the 20th century both early Soviet communism and the secular socialist kibbutz settlements in Israel after 1948 were movements that insisted on the dignity and moral value of all kinds of menial labour undertaken for the common good. Neither movement had any more lasting success than Christianity in undermining the deep-rooted negative status of 'drudgery'. Those demeaning status implications chronically reassert themselves and leave women and low-status men responsible for the hard, menial jobs – the tasks that make the world go round – while providing only meagre, often no, financial rewards and social recognition in return. Lucy Delap describes the nature and status of the domestic labour done by servants: '[It] frequently dealt with tabooed areas of physical existence, to do with the management of dirt and disorder ... tasks not usually done in public' (Delap 2011, p 221). It is unsurprising that first wave suffragists and then second wave feminists from the 1970s onwards found themselves more often outraged by the unequal gender burdens of domestic work than seeking out the hidden (Christian, socialist or communal) virtues of the hard labour of maintenance and care. Delap's comment flags up the need to count the cost when drudgery loses its protective religious carapace and has to be justified in secular, often economic and political, terms.

The drudgery of household labour: women and servants

Patricia Lockwood, a contemporary American poet, novelist and commentator, offers a sardonic feminist slant on the entrenched gender division of household labour. She puts it pithily: 'Most of women's work is what allows life to continue. The rest is like ... Windexing the veneer of civilisation every morning to keep it shiny, or cooking Beef Wellington for a pig king who would be just as happy eating apple cores' (Lockwood 2021, p 10). The historian of domestic service Laura Schwartz lays out the problem that lies behind Lockwood's witty aphorism:

> [L]onger working hours, a diminished welfare state, the need for at least two incomes to adequately support a family, the rise of a global domestic labour market have contributed to a 'crisis of care'. Both women and men are not simply unwilling but often unable to undertake the necessary housework and care for their families. (Schwartz 2019, p 4)

Schwartz begins *Feminism and the Servant Problem* with a summary of our contemporary dilemma, including the reliance on a postcolonial global market for domestic labour, which today recruits some of the poorest on earth to service some of the richest and most fortunate households in the Western world as well as staffing much of the 'care sector' of the welfare state.

It forms the prelude to Schwartz's substantive historical analysis of the way class and gender intersected problematically with the necessities of caring and domestic labour in Britain in the late 19th and early 20th centuries, laying the foundation of our present problems. She treats as axiomatic the tensions over the inclusion of domestic servants that troubled both the women's suffrage movement and the labour movement. For both middle-class suffragists and labour movement organizers, domestic labour was degrading 'drudgery' rather than dignified 'work' and therefore not compatible either with unionized trades or with a feminist work ethic.

There were, perhaps, other considerations at work too, in the difficulties of unionizing domestic servants. In *Labours Lost*, on the role of 18th-century domestic service in England, Carolyn Steedman shows how 18th-century servants were able to appeal to common law and tax law in disputes with their employers over working conditions and remuneration because they were 'inscribed' in the law as individuals and legal persons, so individual cases could be pursued in the courts (Steedman 2009). However, the status of a woman, in law, was less guaranteed than that of a man, and by the 19th century the numerical dominance of females in domestic service was even more pronounced than in the previous century, when male servants had often combined outdoor husbandry with indoor tasks, including such things as childcare, washing or cooking. By the end of the century, when political economy was emerging, trade unions were being founded to provide collective protection for industrial labour that the common law did not afford them as 'corporate persons'.[7] The increasingly female province of domestic work was also seen as problematic within the emerging 'economic' paradigm. Steedman points out that both Adam Smith and Karl Marx regarded domestic service as not the sort of work that warranted inclusion in their analyses of the emerging industrial system (Steedman 2009, p 355). This, perhaps, makes it less surprising that the statesmen, economists and bankers who set up the international financial institutions after the Second World War decided not to include the unpaid domestic work of housewives in new standardized computation of national output, the gross national product, literally rendering women's domestic work officially 'invisible' – unpriced rather than priceless.

Laura Schwartz points out that towards the end of the first decade of the 20th century, when campaigns for female suffrage were at their height, middle-class women involved in the suffrage campaign very seldom paid attention to the position or needs of their domestic servants, even when servants and mistresses stood together in marches and public meetings for the cause (Schwartz 2019). This underlines the habitual asymmetry of attention between servants and their employers. The diaries and letters and the rare autobiographies written by domestic servants reveal how much more notice servants found it necessary to give to the character, habits and priorities of their mistresses than their mistresses ever felt called to reciprocate. Lucy Delap probes this in her study of domestic servants in the 20th century (Delap 2011). She shows how servants had to develop a 'double-consciousness' in their dealings with their employers, recognizing the differences between their often opposed interests and perspectives and knowing that some things could not openly be mentioned in the presence of employers but only aired safely within the 'servants' quarters', though even in that relatively 'private' space the expression was often coded so that it would not easily be understood beyond the servants or even a small inner circle of them. The potential comedy or drama of these divergent views is a persistent theme in literature and popular culture featuring the lives of servants. It is central to the subtleties of Kazuo Ishiguro's bestselling 1989 novel *The Remains of the Day*, later made into a successful film, as well as to the long-lasting appeal of popular comic novels from the interwar period, like P.G. Wodehouse's series featuring the clever valet, Jeeves, and his obtuse master, Bertie Wooster, or Dorothy Sayers' crime novels in which Lord Peter Wimsey draws on the 'know-how' and gossip available to his manservant, Bunter, to supplement what he can glean from his own aristocratic peers. Lucy Delap cites other examples of the role of domestic service in popular culture, showing how double consciousness remains part of the nostalgic attraction of long-running 'country house' costume dramas, such as *Downton Abbey*, which play on the contrasting views from 'upstairs' and 'downstairs' (Delap 2011, pp 206–35).[8] She also notes how the tabooed nature of many of the physical tasks servants undertook, especially dealing with human waste, made it easy to eroticize the servant, for either comic or dramatic effect, in popular culture as well as in real-life relationships of unequal power between employers and their intimate servants. Delap believes this double consciousness is part of the appeal of 'heritage nostalgia', because domestic labour was the source of so many 'untold stories'.

Earlier, we glanced in passing at Virginia Woolf veering unpredictably between wanting to be 'mothered' by her principal woman servant and wanting to be free of the same servant's intrusion into the Woolfs' intimate space. Alison Light recounts the agonies this repeated domestic drama caused, particularly for Woolf's long-serving cook, Nelly Boxall, who was disappointed and resentful at her mistress' failure to offer some personal acknowledgement that might soften the unequal relationship in the intimate setting that was 'home' for the servant as much as for her mistress (Light 2008); Light had originally intended to call the 2008 book *The Problem of Nelly* (Light 2022, pp 134–40, 156–94). Novels of the 19th and 20th centuries suggest much the same asymmetry of attention in what were typically unequal middle- and upper-class marriages, where wives needed to be minutely alert to the needs of husbands, but seldom vice versa. The pattern is not entirely obsolete today.

By the early 20th century, when the domestic dramas of the Woolfs and their servants were being played out, domestic labour had been organized in what Laura Schwartz describes as a routinized timetable of chores resembling the methods of the factory system (Schwartz 2019). Mistresses or their housekeepers often laid out detailed work schedules with few guaranteed rest breaks in a working day of 16 hours or more that made organizing union meetings, attending suffrage rallies or any kind of private life, extremely difficult for resident domestic servants. As late as the 1940s and 1950s, all my older working-class aunts, who had worked in the cotton mill from childhood, imposed a similar routinized system on themselves in their own homes. The schedule of every regular chore for the coming year – cleaning windows, scrubbing steps and paths, scouring cooking stoves, changing beds, washing, ironing, paying the rent, paying the insurance man and so on – was entered in their Co-op calendars before they were hung in the kitchen on New Year's Day and 'religiously' adhered to as the daily, weekly and monthly rhythm of the domestic year unfolded. In her celebrated study of housewives, Ann Oakley found something approximating systematic housework routines and 'standards', usually copied from mothers, was still common among both the working-class and middle-class housewives in her London sample at the beginning of the 1970s (Oakley 1974, 2019). Yet while this method might introduce order into tedious, repeated chores, it was not enough to overcome the dislike of housework common to both the working-class and middle-class housewives in Oakley's sample; almost no one in any social class really enjoys drudgery even if they can appreciate the domestic order it creates.

In *Mrs Woolf and the Servants*, Alison Light devotes a long chapter, with the sardonic title 'Memoirs of a lavatory attendant', to examining Virginia Woolf's attitudes to the labouring classes, especially in the 1930s when she thought she might include some 'low life' scenes in her fiction. Light quotes from Woolf's diaries, notebooks, letters and literary works. Despite having had a rather equivocal friendship with the reformer Margaret Llewelyn Davies, who persuaded her to contribute an introduction to a volume of essays by working women in the Co-operative Women's Guild, Woolf never managed any real imaginative empathy with her lowlier sisters (Light 2008).[9] Light cites examples of Woolf's distaste for the physicality of the rough, heavy work performed by domestic servants and daily 'chars', quoting her often-expressed disgust at their sweat, their servile deference, their intimate connection to dirt, greasy dishcloths, the contents of their masters' and mistresses' chamber pots (even so, she was very reluctant to install a modern bathroom to make the chamber pots redundant). Woolf described their bodies as like 'fat white slugs', one as having a 'large, white, muffin face', and she showed undisguised contempt for their banal chatter and vulgar speech (Light 2008, p 273). Virginia Woolf had an unusually intense distaste for the body as compared to the mind,[10] but her attitudes to the manual labour that fell to the lowest tier of the servant class were broadly shared by many other radical intellectuals as well as by most of the business and professional middle classes who employed them in their homes. It bolstered the employers' confidence in their own superiority and authority.

Just before the Second World War, Virginia Woolf exchanged letters with Agnes Smith, an unemployed wool weaver from Huddersfield who wrote her a long indignant complaint after reading *Three Guineas* in 1938. Agnes Smith was 'irked' by the book and Alison Light quotes from her nine-page letter: 'your book would make some people think that you consider working women, and the daughters of educated men as a race apart. Do you think we enjoy being "hewers of wood and drawers of water", that we do menial tasks from choice and are fitted for nothing else?' (Light 2008, pp 206–7). Smith's account of her own life shows a woman articulate and hungry for education, particularly after a year's course at Hillcroft Adult Education College for Women, but who, like all my mother's older sisters, at age 12 had to go to work in the mill (probably as a 'half-timer'[11]). Smith was unmarried and had to support her mother and sister by doing work for which male weavers were paid 10 per cent above the women's rate and were routinely offered more overtime (Light 2008, p 188 et seq). She wanted Woolf to realize that women's work was rewarded by poverty pay but that 'a working woman who refuses to work will starve'. The correspondence was warm but Woolf never accepted the socialist and feminist views that Agnes Smith had hoped might transform her thinking. Drudgery remained drudgery for Woolf and was, therefore, something for which someone other than 'the daughters of educated men' should take responsibility. She was uncomfortably conscious that her own freedom depended on the work of servants, but her desultory efforts to manage without resident servants involved minimal skill and effort (Light 2008, p 188 et seq). As Francesca Wade puts it: 'The fantasy of living completely without servants never became reality – Woolf's enjoyment of cooking never extended to cleaning' (Wade 2020, p 297). Neither she nor anyone else thought of enrolling her husband, Leonard, to help, though he became an enthusiastic gardener, but for his own satisfaction rather than as 'helping' the gardeners he employed.

Dorothy Sayers was a decade younger than Virginia Woolf, although their social circles marginally overlapped; Sayers even lived for a time in the early 1930s in Mecklenburgh Square, Bloomsbury, where the Woolfs took a flat at the beginning of the Second World War, just in time to be bombed out of it in the Blitz (Wade 2020). Sayers, an Anglican clergyman's daughter, was one of the early women graduates of Somerville College, Oxford, while, like the rest of the intelligentsia, Woolf's affluent family kept her at home and never considered sending a daughter to university alongside her brothers; Woolf habitually claimed she was 'uneducated' and so able to disclaim any responsibility for political problems (Lee 2007, pp 141–5; Light 2022, pp 194–204). Unlike Woolf, Sayers had to earn her living, which included a job writing copy for one of the leading London advertising agencies. She had a successful career in the interwar decades, which continued well into the 1950s, as a bestselling crime novelist, playwright, broadcaster, poet and theologian. Sayers had a more complicated relationship to domestic labour and childcare than the childless Virginia Woolf, but she too struggled over the necessary drudgery and caring tasks that underpin any civilized life but threaten the autonomy, the life of the mind and the career that the 'modern' educated woman aspired to in the 20th century.

One of Sayers' most celebrated crime novels, *Gaudy Night*, published in 1935, is widely regarded as one of the earliest 'feminist' examples of the genre but, more accurately and ambiguously, the novel dramatizes all the contradictions that concern us here. The story is set in a fictional Oxford college for women, plagued by a series of outrages that threaten to harm women's university education. Harriet Vane, Sayers' fictional alter ego, as a crime writer and alumna of the college, is invited to investigate discreetly for the college authorities but has to call in the assistance of Lord Peter Wimsey, whose proposal of marriage she has been fending off for some years as a threat to her independence. The final 'reveal' is only ambiguously 'feminist'. It exposes the perpetrator as a woman servant at the college, a widow working to support two young daughters. She has been employed by the college in a benevolent act, but, as a resident servant, has to pay for her daughters to live as lodgers and be cared for nearby. Her husband had failed his PhD when the woman examiner, who happens to be the newest member of the college, identified a claim he had falsely attributed to an archive source. The husband committed suicide and his widow bore a fierce grudge against women scholars as enemies of male scholars and of 'the domestic woman who only wants the best for her family'. At one level this is a cautionary instance of what Harriet Vane most hates and fears about patriarchal marriage and the kind of blind romantic loyalty that, like the law of evidence at the time, assumes a wife will support her husband, right or wrong. Sayers tries to be even-handed in the novel. Early in the story, after the Gaudy Night dinner, Harriet laments the sad decline into marriage and motherhood of one of the clever friends with whom she had studied, and the waste of her friend's intellectual potential. At the same time she also admires another fellow student who has not allowed marriage and motherhood to impede her career, taking her young family along when she and her husband go on field trips and involving the children in their joint work. Yet, late in the story, Harriet also mistakenly suspects one of the spinster dons of vandalism aimed at Harriet herself, because the austere woman scholar seems to show signs of sexual envy over Lord Peter's attention. At another level, however, the story represents a sharp, feminist critique of the cultural invisibility of wives and domestic servants – only women dons and the students at the college form the 'obvious' pool of suspects, because the servants are seen as no more than their impersonal function and none of the 'educated women' considers for a moment that the culprit might be one of the female servants. Ironically, it is the male sleuth, Wimsey, not the 'feminist' heroine, Harriet Vane, who solves the case, because he is the only person not blinded by the assumption that the servants can have neither independent agency nor interest in the outrage.

Sayers has no real answer to the unpalatable alternatives she lays bare for 'educated' women – marriage, with patriarchal domination and domestic drudgery, or singleness, with, for some, independence, intellectual stimulation and modest financial autonomy, but without motherhood or sexual fulfilment except at the cost of respectability.[12] Sayers simply invents an impossibly perfect fictional man in Peter Wimsey, which allows Harriet Vane to have her cake and eat it, marrying him knowing he will support her writing and treat her as an equal while his fabulous wealth means she need never shoulder the 'drudgery' of childcare and domestic labour – which throws us, and her, right back to 'the servant problem'.

In real life, Sayers found no such magical solution. The men she became involved with, including the irresponsible father of her child and the alcoholic journalist she eventually married, were thoroughly unsatisfactory and sometimes predatory, though they supplied her with good copy for her crime novels. She never told her parents about her illegitimate son but sent him to be fostered by an aunt and cousin whom she paid from her earnings. Sayers only revealed the truth of their relationship to her son well into his adult life. Alison Light takes issue with Barbara Reynolds, Sayers' protégée and biographer, for her sanitized account of Sayers' life, not as the 'sexual deviant, bad mother, heartless wife' of earlier biographical sketches; Light writes: 'Instead of the exuberant, rude and fat eccentric, dramatizing herself and bullying others, she gives us a dreamy young woman, practising a Mona Lisa smile' (Light 2022, p 109). No satisfactory solution except in escapist romantic fantasy, then.[13]

It is intriguing that in the 1980s and 1990s a 'feminist' subtype of crime novel appeared, featuring independent women investigators, some with children, some with semi-detached male or female sexual partners, most with some variety of marginalized status (Munt 1994). For a decade or more, this subgenre enjoyed a substantial readership. As an alternative to Peter Wimsey, and in the spirit of late 20th-century socialist feminism, many of these stories solve the female investigator's problems of poverty, insecurity and/or domestic responsibility by providing her with community support to share the drudgery and childcare or to take over in emergencies, though few are focused quite as directly as Dorothy Sayers' *Gaudy Night* on the way domestic labour and childcare constrain women.

Domestic drudgery in the working-class marital bargain

In *Bread Winner*, Emma Griffin explores the working-class angle on domestic drudgery as compared with that of households that could afford to subcontract it to less fortunate others. Griffin shows the Victorian economy of the domestic household as operating in a quite different way in the working-class households of the industrial North West from how it worked either among the rural labouring classes or in middle-class homes with servants (Griffin 2020). Using a rich cache of autobiographical material from almost 500 manuscripts similar to the account that Agnes Smith sent to Virginia Woolf, Griffin shows that the marital exchange in the families of the labouring classes in industrial towns took distinctive economic form. In agricultural areas, before the Industrial Revolution, the implicit gender bargain in marriage was more equal than it later became in the industrial towns and cities. After the enclosure movement, landless agricultural labourers became entirely dependent on their wives and older children to service the household. Women and children had to gather fuel and often water, and they frequently had to spin the wool they gathered from the hedges and then weave it into cloth to make the family's clothes. Their often rudimentary homes were hard to keep clean in the absence of anything more technologically sophisticated than scraps of material from worn-out garments and brooms with scavenged twigs for heads, and women frequently needed to improvise cleaning aids if soap, beyond the roughest minimum, was unaffordable. Fires were needed for cooking as well as heating and had to be lit very early and tended throughout the day. Some food must be grown or gathered; chickens, pigs, a cow or a goat might need to be kept and eventually slaughtered. In rural areas all food had to be sourced, prepared and cooked by the woman at home as the labourer had no other source of meals. The workload of wives was heavy, and this meant that the care of younger children was largely left to siblings, mainly the older girls. This made compulsory schooling after 1870 (with the Education Act of that year) so difficult for many poor families.

From roughly the mid-19th century, the relative fairness of the marital bargain – male drudgery in the labour market for just enough pay to keep a modest-sized family minimally alive and functioning, in exchange for unremitting domestic drudgery by wives and children, especially daughters – was undermined by two developments in the urban industrial areas. The first was the emergence of an income hierarchy among the male 'breadwinners' in the paid labour market, with skilled artisans earning incomes higher than the subsistence level wages of the rural labourer and of unskilled industrial workers. The second was the appearance of alternative sources of meals outside the home that working men with money at their disposal could use. Initially these consisted largely of cookshops and bakers selling hot food, but later extended to factory canteens, working men's clubs and other commercial outlets. Some men always spent their wages selfishly on themselves, but this was a special temptation for men with above-subsistence incomes. Emma Griffin estimates that around 32 per cent of the food poverty reported in the urban autobiographies she studied, compared with around 10 per cent in the rural ones, was caused by men putting their own priorities before those of the rest of the family. Such male breadwinner needs or pleasures ranged from trades union, friendly society, political party or social club subscriptions to buying books, attending lectures or courses, spending on 'other women' or attending the music hall – but was most often associated with a male culture of heavy drinking (Griffin 2020, p 122). Despite the increased availability and affordability of foodstuffs by the late 19th century, memories of having gone hungry as children remained common right up to the First World War, in some cases even to the mid-1950s. Such chronic child hunger occurred not just because some fathers kept a proportion of their earnings for themselves but also because it was customary to reserve the most nutritious food for the 'breadwinner'; I remember that as still normal in the years of austerity and rationing that continued after the men returned home from the Second World War. Some of the working-class women interviewed in the late 1970s for *Dutiful Daughters* made the same point, occasionally as a complaint about the unfairness of their own childhoods (McCrindle and Rowbotham 1977). Griffin reports that bread was often the main ingredient in Victorian and Edwardian children's meals (Griffin 2020, p 193 et seq). By the 1950s breakfast cereals were supplementing bread in that role.

Much of what had to be done by wives and children in the homes of the labouring classes was performed in middle- and upper-class residences by domiciliary or non-resident servants under the command or supervision of the mistress of the household. In affluent middle-class families, the supervision of the servants might be left to a resident housekeeper, leaving the wife and daughters free to live lives of leisure, or philanthropy or even, among a small intellectual cadre, writing or the arts, though preferably in a respectably 'amateur' fashion. The possibility of status-defining idleness among wives was spreading downwards to lower levels of the middle class who could afford a non-resident 'girl' or a single domestic servant by the late 19th century; Arnold Bennett's parents had eventually reached this pinnacle and Arnold himself acquired a large rural establishment with a fleet of specialist servants at the height of his success around the First World War (Donovan 2022, pp 112–23).

Domestic drudgery: a particular problem for feminists?

Resident domestic servants were no longer part of most business and professional middle-class households by the end of the Second World War, yet the attitudes that discounted or barely noticed the contribution that essential domestic drudgery and childcare made to the household still lurked under, and sometimes above, the surface when the new wave of feminism convulsed the mass media in the late 1960s and 1970s. Some of the new, university-educated feminists hoped the problem might go away if only men would take on half the responsibility for the necessary domestic labour in the home, especially if everyone realized how unnecessary the cult of domestic perfection and women's self-oppressive 'house-proud' attitudes really were – Patricia Lockwood's 'Windexing the veneer of civilisation' and cooking all those beef wellingtons. Women, it was argued, should take full advantage of the labour-saving devices that technological progress was supplying. In her oral history of the British Women's Liberation Movement, Margaretta Jolly quotes Beatrix Campbell scornfully suggesting that the first Ruskin conference of the movement in 1970 was the response of middle-class mothers to 'servantless' homes (Jolly 2019, p 21). Bea Campbell, an early historian of the movement, herself from a working-class communist family in Carlisle, took an uncompromising socialist feminist position, although in conversation with Margaretta Jolly for *Sisterhood and After* she admitted that her initial response had perhaps been an oversimplification (Jolly 2019, p 21). Her retraction should not be taken to mean there was no substance to her barb; it was a shrewd observation of the middle-class character and implicit assumptions of much of second wave feminism.

Accounts of that first Ruskin conference, an offshoot of the Ruskin History Workshop, make a point of mentioning that the male partners of some of the women manned the creche while the women got on with debating and agitating. The men included Stuart Hall, the Jamaican-born sociologist who founded the Birmingham Centre for Cultural Studies and was the husband of the historian Catherine Hall; and Raphael Samuel, who taught at Ruskin, was the genius loci of the History Workshop and at that time the partner of feminist community historian Anna Davin, and co-carer of her children (Jolly 2019; Light 2019). Both women had been part of the organizing committee of the conference. Yet Margaretta Jolly also records the guffaws of many of the men in the History Workshop when the idea of that first Women's Liberation meeting was mooted (Jolly 2019, p 26).

The question of who should do all that necessary care and drudgery has for long been a problem for feminism, as Bea Campbell's immediate response to that first Ruskin conference might suggest. Lucy Delap makes a similar judgement: 'Post-war feminists proved inadequately attentive to the disadvantages of class and ethnicity experienced by those women to whom domestic work was still delegated', illustrating her point through the naive fantasy of Germaine Greer in her 1970 bestseller *The Female Eunuch* of advocating collective living in an Italian farmhouse where all the domestic chores and gardening would be done by 'a local family who lived in the house' (Delap 2011, p 131). The socialist feminist tradition that Bea Campbell represents, was inclined to favour collective households that could share all chores among the members and take advantage of economies of scale that pooling resources made possible, and to agitate for state funding of nurseries, high-quality childcare and improved housing provision. The stifling 'privacy' of the bourgeois family might be mitigated, and the increasing isolation of wives and mothers in the mobile 'nuclear family' reversed, by such arrangements. In fact, communal households were always a small minority, even among committed feminists. Yet, a telling phrase in Jolly's oral history highlights the intimate mutual bonding of the sisterhood that could be sharply jolted when race and class differences within the movement were brutally exposed. Jolly quotes the argument of Nathalie Thomlinson that 'part of the psychological shock white women felt over being challenged on race' could be attributed to 'the small group structure and *intense ethic of care* within the WLM [Women's Liberation Movement], which led many women to expect self-valorization alongside taking on each other's traumas' (Jolly 2019, p 182, emphasis added). This looks like a transmutation of the feminization not of piety but of care itself into a feminist secular modality as 'sisterhood'.

Sex, family, drudgery and care as feminist concerns

Aspects of middle-class feminism from the 1960s and 1970s focused on issues such as combatting widespread sexual ignorance, releasing female sexual pleasure from the taboos that controlled and inhibited it, demonstrating the oppressive nature of the nuclear family and patriarchal power, and recognizing the isolation, frustration and monotony of being a full-time housewife, especially in anonymous modern suburbia, notably for the new cohort of 'educated women'. Each of the different elements in this list has its own research and polemical literature. The issue of female sexuality probably got most exposure in the mass media for its titillation value, but also achieved a wider distribution of knowledge not only about female orgasm but about gynaecological health, methods of contraception, postnatal medical complications and the prevalence of female depression. The housewives in Ann Oakley's research and the housebound young mothers of Hannah Gavron's pioneering study, *The Captive Wife*, were discontented with the life of a 'housewife', irrespective of their class background: the sheer grind of housework was disliked pretty universally (Gavron 1966; Oakley 1974).

But as Lucy Delap shrewdly notes, Hannah Gavron had seen the discontent of middle-class 'captive wives' as lying, at least in part, in realizing that their situation was no better than that of working-class housewives (Delap 2011, p 131). Delap's summary of the situation in the first decades after the Second World War reads: 'The housewife did not appear as a settled identity willingly embraced by post-war women but rather as a problematic subject position into which middle-class women from formerly servant-keeping families had been forced' (Delap 2011, p 132). Delap sees the class grievance of middle-class housewives in servantless households as the root of subsequent radicalization of attitudes to the gendering of domestic labour, a conclusion not so different from Bea Campbell's spontaneous verdict in 1970.

Class and ethnicity: fault lines in feminism?

Among the fault lines that potentially divided the feminist movement, the class difference was always crucial, and activism among working-class women was more usually channelled into trade union disputes and strikes over working conditions, demands for equal pay and demands for state-supported childcare rather than into issues focused narrowly on the burden of domestic labour for women. Ethnic identity, or 'race', like class, had a powerful salience which, again, often showed itself in industrial disputes, especially in the 1970s and 1980s, and in instances where ethnic minority women made common cause with their menfolk against what were criticized as privileged White feminist attacks on men's supposed universal propensity for toxic violence and their assumptions of entitlement. This, it was argued, demonstrated the blindness of White middle-class feminists to the class and race dimensions of gender inequality. This approach has much in common with Kenan Malik's (2023) critique of how intersections of class and 'race' bedevilled the Labour movement. Margaretta Jolly's oral history of the Women's Liberation Movement in Britain gives a careful account of these and other chronic divisions (Jolly 2019, pp 25–34, 133, 159–203, 244). Analysis of the 'intersectionality' of different structures or cultures of division, discrimination or disadvantage, such as race, class, gender or sexuality, has become a more prominent feature of attempts to theorize the complex interactions between these elements, particularly in 21st-century feminist scholarship.[14] It is, nevertheless, possible to use the concept of intersectionality to suggest that one dimension of 'power' can partly compensate for the disadvantages of another, rather than automatically intensifying inequality in all the dimensions of power.[15]

The new wave of feminism in the 1960s and 1970s often appeared anarchic, with single-issue campaigns crosscut with all kinds of Left political groupings with liberal and libertarian impulses that had contradictory political implications. Critiques of the way 'bourgeois' or 'patriarchal' marriage and traditional domestic burdens exploited and disadvantaged women were part of the weave. Ever since Eleanor Rathbone had criticized the tradition of 'the male breadwinner', and, for reasons made clear by Emma Griffin's research, had campaigned to put part of the family income directly into the hands of the woman (Griffin 2020), feminists and social reformers had begun to document the 'invisible' and unpaid caring and domestic labour undertaken routinely by women. When a proposal that wages should be paid to women for their 'invisible' housework emerged in the 1970s, feminists were far from unified over it, not least over who, realistically, would pay these wages. One eventual offshoot of this concern was The Women's Budget Group, which started work in the early 1990s gathering evidence of exactly what was necessary to enable women to manage the household economy, especially in disadvantaged and female-headed families. The group, a feminist think-tank, has been an ongoing resource for policy making, though the actual use made of its research and arguments by politicians has been very uneven.

Underpinning most feminist thinking since the 1960s has been a determination to unravel sex and gender stereotypes (or 'constructs' or 'discourses') to reveal them as cultural rather than primarily 'natural' or biological programmes and therefore open to challenge and change. It is telling that while there were heated disagreements within the feminist movement about whether 'motherhood' was or was not a biological drive that made it 'natural' for every mother to bond with her newborn child (though not all do, in reality), and disputes over whether women were 'naturally' carers, there were no parallel arguments about whether an instinct for domestic hard labour was built into female biology – it does not obviously enhance a woman's sexual desirability to insist on her 'natural' prowess with the scrubbing brush, the washing up bowl or the ironing board. Nobody, it seems, wants to claim drudgery as their 'natural' right. Within a common effort to expose the cultural construction of gender inequality, a range of different feminist preoccupations emerged piecemeal as specific grievances were experienced as urgent by particular groups of women. Household drudgery was only one of them, and it had variable resonance and priority across class and ethnicity.

At the end of her book on housework, Ann Oakley moves from a carefully calibrated, 'objective', 'scientific' approach to social research as a value-neutral fact-finding exercise to admit the value-saturated issue of what her findings 'mean' for the cause of women's liberation (Oakley 1974). Most of the housewives she interviewed were either indifferent or hostile to the Women's Liberation Movement, even though they had many common dissatisfactions with the role of housewife and complaints about the greater freedom of husbands. In a later edition, Oakley argues that her data suggest that this apparent contradiction is explained by 'the tendency among housewives towards a strong psychological identification with conventional definitions of femininity'; gender stereotypes are so deeply embedded that only 'consciousness-raising' in women-only groups can make inroads into them (Oakley 2019, p 185). The new introduction Oakley wrote for the 2019 reissue of the book makes clear that precious little had changed in the half-century since the first edition. She summarizes:

> Gender ideology continues to act as a powerful driver of behaviour. If women's immersion in housework is to reduce, both quantitatively and qualitatively, the responsibility needs to be shared. Yet this requires the dissolution of men's resistance to change, a resistance which is irresistibly bolstered by beliefs in housework as a female domain. Answers to the same survey questions over two decades yield very limited evidence of change in women's and men's share of unpaid domestic and care work … . Women remain more likely to consider the gender division of domestic labour unfair, and men to hold resolutely to the belief that they do enough. (Oakley 2019, p xi)

For Oakley and other feminists, this is a reason to find ways to change the feminine stereotype, even though the resistance of men to doing more domestic labour is a chronic brake on change. Yet, as Laura Schwartz reminds us, neither men nor women have time or energy left over from their paid employment to do it all (Schwartz 2019). Even with a more gender-equal distribution of necessary drudgery, the obvious solution seems to be to subcontract it to less privileged folk, such as servants historically were, which poses its own moral, economic and political problems – and/or to get state support.

Lessons from feminist memoirs: nurturing, nesting, drudgery and care

Recent memoirs of second wave feminists from the 1960s and 1970s are a rich source of information about the contradictions they encountered over the distribution of the inevitable quota of drudgery and the solutions they tried out. Because they are based on personal recollections, diaries and letters, these memoirs are often more illuminating than formal studies about the things that may not appear in the index of a research report but that act as tripwires in the exigencies of everyday life. Sheila Rowbotham's memoirs, for instance, are vivid accounts of the maelstrom of the period among many varieties of feminists (Rowbotham 2021). She juggled efforts to unionize women night cleaners in London offices and personal struggles to reconcile sexual freedom and non-possessive relationships with a desire for long-term commitments and shared childrearing, while also earning an independent living by freelance teaching and writing. Rowbotham is particularly revealing on parenthood and the way biology can ambush a feminist in defiance of her ideological convictions and intentions. Feminists had been outraged by the idea that all women have inbuilt maternal instincts and are 'naturally' monogamous, while men are 'naturally' polygamous and lacking a biological drive for childcare. Mary Harrington, the self-styled 'reactionary feminist' whose ideas featured in the previous chapter, goes as far as suggesting that second wave feminism was split between the alternative priorities of freedom or care (Harrington 2023). An illustration of the divided mind of feminism was seen in reactions to the second thoughts of noted American feminist Alice Rossi. In the 1970s, Rossi admitted she had underestimated biological differences in the relative importance of parenthood for women and men. Her change of mind created widespread outrage among feminists such as Ann Oakley, who saw it as a denial of the power of cultural construction in what they believed was wrongly accepted as 'natural' (Oakley 1974). Now, in the 2020s, revisionist feminists such as Mary Harrington and Louise Perry reassert the 'natural' character of biological sexual difference and the importance of women caring for their own children (Perry 2022; Harrington 2023).

The feminist movement's split mind can already be glimpsed back in the early days of its second wave. Sheila Rowbotham and her then partner, Paul Atkinson, decided to have a child in the 1970s and to share the childcare equally. When she became pregnant, she began to notice how much more 'immediate and material' issues that had seemed abstract became for her, particularly those concerned with childcare provision and childcare workers. She was astonished by the strength of her nurturing feelings toward her son when he was born, much as Harrington was two generations later when her daughter was born. On one occasion, while Rowbotham was delivering a lecture, her attention was distracted by catching sight of her baby son in his father's arms at the back of the room. She recalls: 'Mothering and Identity were beginning to look more tricky than I had bargained for' (Rowbotham 2021, p 234). The kickback of the biological can be fierce and unexpected, particularly, perhaps, for some convinced feminist 'constructionists'.

Most of Ann Oakley's sample of housewives in the late 1960s found childcare more satisfying than housework. Some of their dislike of routine, repetitive household chores was related to the way unpredictably urgent needs of childcare could disrupt the housework schedule, and vice versa. Although it was not without its problems, most of Oakley's housewives found real pleasure in childcare, particularly dressing their children nicely when they took them out. Oakley interprets this as evidence of the strength of the stereotype of femininity that they have culturally absorbed (Oakley 2019, p 151). Yet it is striking that among men who do try to take their share of domestic responsibility, one of the most favoured roles is spending time caring for and playing with children – in fact, the 'fun bits' of parenting as distinct from the grind of repetitive cleaning and maintenance or the responsibility for routinely planning necessary chores. But fun is often inextricable from drudgery. Even changing babies' nappies is an opportunity for intimate play, including singing games and the like. One of the best descriptions I know of the joys of early childcare was written by a man who describes his delight in recent fatherhood. The journalist, writer and therapist, Matthew McNaught, writes:

> I was grateful for the moments of sheer delight alongside the stress and drudgery. These were less of a surprise than the quiet satisfaction of the drudgery itself. Sleep-deprived and unkempt hanging out at the soft play on a Saturday as L explored. I felt diminished and extended, at once less alive and more alive than I'd ever felt before. As tyrannical as parenthood could sometimes be, one of its gifts was that it demanded neither originality nor excellence. You only had to turn up to be a servant of the superorganism. To clean, to change, to soothe. To sing the nursery rhymes, or rather let them sing through you, strange immortal creatures that they are. To get down on your knees on the linoleum of the kitchen floor for the nightly ritual: picking up, one by one, the sweetcorn and the peas. (McNaught 2022, p 136)

McNaught captures perfectly the difficulty of separating the drudgery from the joy in caring for children. He was writing a book at home, an elastic process so far as timing goes, when he wrote that aside on the rigours and joys of parenthood. It pinpoints the exhausting but exhilarating parental experience at the point in a child's life where fundamental bonding and security are built, a process that works both ways in the relationship. As a writer, his working day at that juncture did not involve showing up at a place of work and could accommodate sleep deprivation and fatigue for a limited time. By contrast, in the 1970s, Sheila Rowbotham, who, like McNaught, was a freelance lecturer and writer, was not prepared for the consequence of sharing childcare equally with Paul Atkinson. It meant that neither of them was 'economically viable' even with intermittent assistance with their son's care from various friends. Theirs was an unanticipated encounter with the problem summarized by Laura Schwartz. A modern political economy expects both men and women to have paid employment but does not adequately fund welfare services to replace the 'invisible' labour of sustaining home and family – housework, childcare, eldercare, care for the sick and disabled. It follows that, even in the utopian position that Rowbotham and Atkinson had agreed, where drudgery and care work are no longer gendered, they were unable to do all the work of maintenance that came with having a child without a potentially disastrous decline in income for their insecure work. Ann Oakley's recipe of getting men to do their full share simply was not enough to solve the problem. Moreover, Rowbotham and Atkinson lived in different collective households and she comments how much more systematically the women organized domestic chores than the men did – the men never seemed to get round to the washing up – and how much more comfortable the women generally made their shared house. The female duty of 'care', it seems, includes cultivating domestic comfort, and whether it is 'constructed' or 'instinctual', it is astonishingly deep-rooted.

Alison Light's touching memoir of her marriage to Raphael Samuel in the late 1980s is full of vivid details about the role of household labour in the very different lives the marriage united, just as one might expect from someone who has written with such insight about the lives of servants (Light 2019). Light calls herself 'the Portsmouth girl who had lost her footing in her own class', the working class, largely through education and the radical politics she met when reading English at Sussex University. She describes her grandmother, who had been in service, being caustic about 'those who did not know one end of a broom from another', and identifies her as the source of the family's domestic habits and exacting housework standards (Light 2019, p 131). Light's ten-year marriage to Raphael Samuel, which ended with his early death in 1997, introduced her into a radically unfamiliar social milieu. They lived in a ramshackle 18th-century house in Spitalfields (since their time, thoroughly gentrified) which was then owned by Samuel but shared promiscuously with the History Workshop as an ever-open meeting place, library and archive, meaning none of its spaces was 'private'. Samuel's was an old communist family that had raised him in collective living while Light's working-class family had conventionally left housework and childcare to the women while reserving certain heavy jobs for the men. Light says her new husband 'boggled at my household lore', something as simple as wiping crumbs from the table into her hand rather than sweeping them on to the floor; 'No doubt we did the minimum by most people's standards' (Light 2019, pp 130–131). Yet she felt connected through her domestic culture to her mother and grandmother and used it to create small enclaves of relative privacy and order of a kind that she found comfortingly familiar among the disconcerting bohemian communal chaos.[16] 'Once I had moved in properly, cleaning and tidying – all the rituals of domesticity – were a way of feeling at home', she writes (Light 2019, p 130 et seq). She bought a new, more efficient cooker and comfortable furniture and curtains for 'the room' in which she and Raphael slept: 'I carried on home-making, improving', she writes. Her husband admired her 'domestic culture' which he saw as evidence of her politically admirable willingness to do the tasks usually left, parasitically, to the lower orders. He joined in enthusiastically but 'preferred the labour intensive' – sweeping, scrubbing lavatories and floors, for instance – and cooking for anyone who happened to be in the house, but never remotely reaching Light's grandmother's standards of order and cleanliness (Light 2019, pp 131, 132, 135–136). Her memoir is a tender depiction of the odd but loving coalescence of two radically different cultures of domestic labour in a household where such matters were subordinate to writing, intellectual community and political life but which disdained to subcontract drudgery to less 'important' other people. On that, the two were entirely at one. Light says 'I was surprised to learn how many feminists, past and present, employed cleaners as a matter of course, never asking their menfolk to do chores but happy to delegate their dirty work to other women' (Light 2019, p 130).

Like the Woolfs, Light and Samuel had no children, so they never had to confront the emotionally and logistically complex problems of reconciling childcare and professional work that ambushed Rowbotham and Atkinson. When I married, I had taken parental responsibility for a stepson and then had three further children. I quickly encountered dilemmas about how to reconcile my academic life with childcare and domestic labour. I tried to avoid loading crushing burdens of housework and childcare on to my severely anxious and overstretched husband (who had several periods of hospital treatment for anxiety and stress in the 1970s and early 1980s). I employed local women to help with the children and they swiftly became quasi-family. I also gratefully accepted the one day a week when my in-laws took over, but like Alison Light, I never felt it right to employ someone else to do the drudgery. So I compromised my standards, bore the silent reproof of my mother-in-law, ran myself ragged trying to do everything, and blamed myself for my failures, never admitting that I was trying to do the impossible. Research time and sleep inevitably suffered. My creativity was never in the same league as Christina Rossetti's or Maeve Gilmore's, but I did write a journal article '"Mother wouldn't like it!" Housework as magic', which attempted to explain how the rituals of housework secured symbolic and even a measure of actual control over the ever-threatening domestic chaos of home and family life for otherwise 'powerless' women, and to acknowledge, as Alison Light does, the unfashionable but real satisfaction of creating distinctively working-class islands of domestic order (Martin 1984).[17] It was not a 'feminist' argument but it made a different kind of sense of the way women use their oppressions as resources of sectoral power that gives them a measure of pride and dignity. I felt it important to make a case for all my female forbears who had done just that in far more intractable situations than mine. It took me a very long time to recognize the truth of what Laura Schwartz puts so succinctly and to conclude that it should be a problem for public policy rather than individual families alone to solve.

The current problem of domestic labour

The pragmatic verdict arrived at by generations of 'educated women' after my own lies behind Laura Schwartz's diagnosis and Mary Harrington's revisionist feminist fury: that without radical changes in economic and welfare policies, women must choose between high-flying careers and raising children. From around 1970, professional women began to postpone or avoid marriage, put off childbearing until the last possible point in their fertile years or reject it altogether. One consequence of the trend to postpone childbirth is that middle-class grandmothers are now on average older than in earlier generations and are sometimes still in paid work. Many of them established their own careers after a break, or slowdown, for childcare, and they are often now caring for their parents. As the sitcom *Motherland* (2016–22) depicts it, they are unwilling to sacrifice to grandchild care the first time in their own lives when they have leisure to please themselves. Moreover, full-time jobs today demand ever more of the worker's efforts and commitment as employers chase increased 'productivity'. Most households today need two incomes, and women are far more likely than men to work part time, either in the job they trained for or, not infrequently, in occupations for which they are overqualified, in order to have time and energy for household labour and childcare. Hence Laura Schwartz's conclusion: 'both women and men are not only unwilling but unable to undertake the necessary housework and care for their families' (Schwartz 2019, p 4). Schwartz goes further, pointing to the recruitment of a global workforce to make up the shortfall.

A new servant class to solve the care crisis?

Lucy Delap (2011, p 127) shows that in the first decades of postwar austerity in the mid-20th century, the servant class virtually disappeared, but by the 1980s it re-emerged in a new form, including a sector of residential domestic workers sourced from abroad, but also new British entrepreneurs, many of them women, who set up small private companies to provide cleaning and childcare services to overstretched households.[18] The renewed 'servant class' began with au pairs and 'mothers' helps' who were often from middle-class families from abroad. Delap argues that this compromised the authority of employers, especially where employers came from families that had never kept servants. Between the 1980s and the present day, a global market for domestic and all forms of care work has emerged by which people from poor and undeveloped economies take on much of the drudgery that was once the lot of the lower orders in Britain. They often do so because there is no work for them or even lower levels of pay or little hope of advancement in their own societies. The global trade in drudges can also include people trafficked for the purpose as part of modern slavery, along with recruitment to agricultural gangs and prostitution (Oakley 2019, pp xii, 29, 213). This global labour force can be paid less than would be necessary to recruit labour to these jobs from the existing British labour force. This is a chronic problem for the social care sector in Britain in the 2020s and also affects recruitment to nursing and healthcare in the NHS. Successive British governments have 'solved' it by encouraging more labour migration to bridge the gap. Families back home often depend on the income repatriated by such migrants, but this migration clearly 'poaches' labour and skills from poorer countries, which usually have an need to build their own health and social care capacity. Alongside the fact that, historically, these forms of employment have been seen as 'women's work', this can depress the levels of remuneration and status in the domestic and care sector of the British economy and exacerbate the contemporary 'crisis of care', to which I now turn.

7

The Care Crisis

The components of care and their ethical rationale

I begin with two glimpses of the care crisis, from the outside and from the inside. They give a clear pointer to the size and urgency of what we face. In the first, Rory Stewart (soldier, diplomat, writer, academic, ex-MP and founder of the Turquois Mountain charity in Afghanistan) describes his walk through Cumbria when he was first preparing to stand as Conservative candidate for Penrith and the Border in the 2010 election (Stewart 2023). He was shocked by the standards in the local hospital, which, for example, had a very poor cancer survival rate, and by the generally inadequate social care he found among the needy people in the predominantly rural area of the constituency.

> The number of people with Alzheimer's in the constituency had doubled in fifteen years. Twice on my walk I knocked on a door and, after a long wait, found a man in a dressing gown, barely competent, who invited me into a house with the smell of food uncleared, and nappies undisposed of. Old people were entitled to see a carer for only fifteen minutes a day – hardly time to wash them, certainly not time to chat. None of the parties seemed willing to tackle this problem. It felt as though the communities I had worked with in Kabul looked after their elderly better than we did in Britain. (Stewart 2023, p 47)

Stewart served as MP for the constituency between 2010 and 2019 and as a member of the Conservative Cabinet for most of that time. He stood unsuccessfully in the election of 2019 for the leadership of the Party after Theresa May resigned, and later that year he was expelled from the Party and deselected as MP by text along with 20 other prominent critics of the new leader, Boris Johnson, and his hard Brexit policy. Rory Stewart now hosts a popular political podcast jointly with Alastair Campbell who had been Director of Communications in the Tony Blair government. Neither of the governments they served managed to tackle the increasingly urgent care crisis.

My second glimpse of that crisis comes from Penny Wincer, an interiors and lifestyle photographer who describes some of the problems of people like herself who find themselves responsible for a relative with a high level of need (Wincer 2020). When it became clear that her severely autistic son needed 24-hour care, she found she was entitled to limited paid help. She cut down her professional work, became a blogger and media activist on behalf of home carers and wrote the eloquent account of her own and other unpaid carers' stressful lives in the book from which the following passage is taken.

> Though some people may wish the role of carer had never fallen on their shoulders … the responsibility of supporting someone they love has given them a sense of purpose and pride … . That's not to say that most carers aren't desperate for more support … . There is also the matter of up to 700,000 young carers in the UK who do an estimated £12,000 of caring each year. Caring that should be being provided by social services, not young children. (Wincer 2020, pp 247–8)

As we have seen throughout this whole analysis, there is more than one way of representing what 'care' is, just as there is of deciding who has a 'duty of care' and to whom that duty is owed; and few of them can appropriately be assigned a market price or organized humanely or efficiently purely through a market mechanism. In a review of Laura Schwartz's *Feminism and the Servant Problem*, Alison Light comments with characteristic insight and economy on some fundamental difficulties:

> comparisons across time, across sectors and between cleaning and other forms of carework are tricky. … [C]are as a social value needs another set of arguments – moral and ethical. But it also needs another language, in order to explore our relations to the body, to helplessness in infancy and age, to our waste products. The concept of work stretches only so far. (Light 2020, p 23)

One object of this chapter is to raise the moral and ethical problems and the political and economic choices posed by our individual and collective responsibility for our fellow human beings over the whole gamut of 'care' in a rapidly changing context of demography, economics, technology and the structures of work. For very many employed women, this care and household labour is what Arlie Hochschild memorably called 'the second shift' of their working lives (see Hochschild and Machung 1989).

I begin with the porous boundary between care and cleaning that Alison Light identifies and with which we are already very familiar. A mixture of childcare and cleaning (drudgery) has usually been the main responsibility of women in the household, and they generally find childcare more rewarding than cleaning. Looking after children is unequivocally 'care' to most people, yet it encompasses many things that involve cleaning the body and dealing with its detritus as well as the material mess typically created by children's activities; that is undoubtedly 'work'. But the whole ensemble is recognized as 'care' because an emotional and practical concern for our children is understood as a normal and necessary part of being a parent. We do, after all, call it child*care* as against house*work*. To complicate matters, it is often in cleaning and tending to the bodies of our children that we build up the first, foundational, intimate bonds with them, particularly if something like feeding children, changing a nappy, bathing or dressing them for bed is lightened with rhymes, stories, chat or all kinds of physical fun. That is true of parenting by any gender: we saw it in the passage from Matthew McNaught in the previous chapter, describing his mixture of exhaustion and exhilaration when taking care of his first child.

Being a carer for variously disabled, old, frail or sick adults and children entails the same kind of intertwined care and labour, whether the care is undertaken by a relative or by a paid worker, although the relative proportions of care and drudgery vary hugely. This ambiguous entanglement was highlighted by the reaction of a member of the audience to an account that my son gave at a public meeting in an English cathedral about working as a carer a few years after disabling illness had put an end to his career in social care. He explained what was involved in caring for adults with severe learning disabilities as well as serious physical impairments at the specialist day centre where he had worked. He set out the problems, for example, in safely giving the clients their regular medicines, in using hoists to get them on and off the lavatory, cleaning their bodies, helping them eat, taking them on outings and activities, getting their motorized wheelchairs safely into the van and securing them for the journey, and getting them out at the other end. He stressed the carer's continual concern for the dignity of clients and the need to stay alert for any signs of physical or emotional distress, or of pleasure, in the restricted body language of clients who typically had little or no speech or mobility. At the end of his talk, a member of the audience exclaimed: 'But it must be very satisfying!' My son's response was: 'Yes. Sometimes. But 99 per cent of what carers do is sheer hard grind.' Much of the gratification is moral and often retrospective, particularly when they care for people whose ability to express appreciation or friendliness is seriously restricted – carers may be left in the dark about whether their clients enjoyed helping to prepare and cook lunch or the special visit to the 'sensory pod' or the warm pool, or if they maybe just endured it all. The relation between carer and cared-for is not always the mutual exchange of affection and tenderness that is sometimes sentimentally projected onto it by people who have directly experienced neither side of such a relationship. It is often hard for carers in the sort of work my son used to do to get a reliable sense of whether they are doing a good job for their clients or to detect any reciprocity, however much the worker may care about the client's dignity, comfort and wellbeing. In this part of the care sector, it takes time and experience to learn to read the often-oblique responses as well as requiring considerable physical strength and a high tolerance of ambiguity, frustration and unsavoury tasks.

In James Butler's brief, incisive diagnosis of the current care crisis, he makes the same observation: that care work can take brutal effort and needs a strong stomach to cope with the feel and smells of the body's waste products (Butler 2023). Butler draws on the 2021 article by Andrew Key in an online magazine about sleep-in shifts in residential care. A judgement of the English Supreme Court in March 2021 rejected the claim of care workers that overnight 'sleep-ins' in residential care settings should be paid at least minimum wage rates. The Court decreed that they are not 'work' and therefore do not qualify for any pay. Key, a novelist and former care worker, is outraged at this judgement, given his own experience of the anxiety generated by that kind of 'wired' night when the carer has to be alert for potential problems even during what is supposed to be rest and sleep. Key is scathing about well-intentioned sentimentality of the kind my son encountered at his talk, what Butler calls 'a weakly secularized Christian caritas'. Butler quotes Key making much the same point as my son: 'The love I feel in fleeting bursts at work is painful and complicated' (Butler 2023, p 14).

Accounts by carers show the standard economic definition of carework as 'unskilled' is a travesty. The human value of such indispensable, emotionally, psychologically and physically demanding interpersonal work cannot be caught in the sort of scale that defines accountancy, financial expertise, business management or scientific research as 'skilled', because it requires a particular set of cerebral activities or high-level academic qualifications. Like other 'people-facing' work, caring calls, above all, on human attributes such as empathy, kindness, patience, humour and tolerance – very much the virtues St Paul ascribed to Christian love, or *agape* – rather than requiring rare technical or intellectual accomplishments or lending itself to measures of increased productivity – doing caring tasks faster is usually not more efficient but less caring, since it is time and attention that the person being cared for mostly needs. To be sure, carers need training in such skills as safely lifting or moving the bodies of those they care for without harming themselves or the person they are caring for; they may benefit from knowing sign language or studying what is known about different kinds of disability and about government policies, and so on. Economists do not need to go as far as consulting St Paul's Epistles; they need only consider the importance Adam Smith, the father of their discipline, attributed to 'moral sentiments' as the invisible underpinning of any properly functioning market system and, most of all, of the structures of trust on which it depends. Applying the usual economic measures does violence to the human value of the work we call 'care'.

State and family in the provision of home care: unequal partners

The problems for care workers touched on earlier are different only in degree and duration for people caring for sick, old or disabled relatives at home, with or without help from professional care workers. Frances Young, Penny Wincer, Margaret Spufford and Eva Feder Kittay have all written about this experience with their disabled children (Spufford 1989; Kittay 2002; Young 2014; Wincer 2020). They testify to times when they were unable to understand what was causing the sometimes extreme and unassuageable distress of their children, or find how to soothe it, despite all their love and patience. The comedy drama series *There She Goes* (2018–) airs these difficult issues lightly and so successfully that it has been given repeat showings on the BBC. Yet these carers also celebrate the joy of reciprocity in the relationship. Carers for spouses or older relatives suffering from dementia often make the same point, even when the person receiving care no longer remembers who the carer is. Caring for parents may also bring the awkward piquancy of a generational inversion of the care relationship. This is part of the dynamic that Emily Kenway describes in her account of four exhausting and distressing years caring for her dying mother: in her book, she intersperses her own experiences with vignettes showing the problems faced by other carers that frequently push them to the verge of despair and exhaustion (Kenway 2023). When the care is given by paid strangers, mutual emotional exchange can be harder to find, particularly when the carer has not had a continuous experience of the client, when they are only one of a frequently changing team that the disabled or sick person never really has time to get to know personally, when the disability of the person needing care is such that reciprocity is difficult to express or when the carer is severely limited by a tight time schedule. Squeezed timetables are increasingly common in Britain's severely underfunded and understaffed social care sector, as Rory Stewart found. Penny Wincer also notes how having to 'rush through' work, such as getting people up and dressing them before the next scheduled appointment, means that paid agency carers have no time to take account of the 'preferences and the emotional needs' of those for whom they are caring (Wincer 2020, p 205).

Emma Dowling makes the case even more sharply and politically. She argues that the imperatives of increasing productivity, reducing labour costs, and protecting the profits of the private companies to which much of social care has been outsourced since the 1980s, has had the effect of steadily reducing 'care' to its 'labour' component – that is, the practical tasks that can be measured and timed and so used as an index of 'productivity'. This comes at the expense of less tangible and unmeasurable but essential human aspects of 'care'. Dowling writes:

> As care work is redefined as the physical provision of support and assistance, the affective, relational and emotional dimensions of caring are increasingly relegated to unpaid realms. Thus, in addition to the stresses and strains of tighter time controls on care workers, what we see … is that even as the job of caring is made more difficult by the measures imposed, the system relies on the fact that care workers continue to care despite all this. In effect, homecare workers' compassion and sense of responsibility are enlisted in order to keep homecare services functioning. (Dowling 2022, p 121)

This last point applies with even more force to relatives, like Penny Wincer and Emily Kenway, who occupy the default position when it comes to who should be responsible for care and who is expected to provide the emotional and relational 'unpaid care' that the state increasingly shuffles off to the 'private' sphere even when it does fund some paid care. In most cases, the state assumes a relative will do the caring unless and until the family officially requests help. Even when these requests are successful, the situation remains perilous for the 'responsible relative', who will often have other responsibilities – a job, other children or adult dependants – particularly as so many marital partnerships collapse under the burden of caring for a disabled child or other kin. Penny Wincer observes that it is common for relatives to have to spend enormous amounts of time finding substitutes for paid carers who cancel at the last moment, or having to drop their own plans, which can include their paid employment. She adds:

> With the social care system buckling under the weight of ten years' worth of government cuts, there is simply not enough money to go around. At the moment everyone – including those who have terminal illness, life-long, untreatable conditions and progressive conditions with no chance of recovery – is forced into being continually re-assessed for their eligibility for social care. These assessments can be invasive and extremely stressful for both the person who needs care and their family members. Many people will let themselves be burned out administering the care themselves rather than rely on social care that can be taken away at any time. (Wincer 2023, p 204)

Like Frances Young, the American feminist philosopher, Eva Feder Kittay was confronted by the problem when she gave birth to a severely disabled child who had no prospect of a 'normal' life. Both Young and Kittay found that it was difficult to justify public support for such disabled 'citizens' under prevalent forms of political and moral philosophy that rest on utilitarian calculations or on liberal notions of a 'social contract' between 'rational' individuals (Kittay 2002; Young 2014). Kittay gravitated to a secular theory of social justice. Over 20 years ago, when Kittay wrote the essay to which I refer, she used the term 'severely retarded' to describe people with brain damage similar to that of her daughter (Kittay 2002, p 268), a usage that would today be avoided as discriminatory. This change of terminology perhaps indicates an increased sensitivity about disability even if it does not reflect much improvement in care or funding. Yet, Kittay's fundamental point remains valid: whatever label we give them, the severely learning disabled tend to act as the 'limiting case' of the category of persons the state deems to deserve its care and therefore its funding. Kittay counters thinking that sets the severely learning disabled apart from the 'normal' majority by pointing out our universal state of dependence and interdependence:

> Independence, except in some particular actions and functions, is a fiction, regardless of our disabilities, and the pernicious effects of this fiction are encouraged when we hide the ways in which our needs are met in relations of dependencies. On the other hand, this fiction turns those whose dependence cannot be masked into pariahs or makes them objects of disdain or pity ... . In acknowledging dependency we respect the fact that as individuals our dependency relations are constitutive of who we are and that, as a society, we are inextricably dependent on one another. (Kittay 2002, p 268)

Kittay argues for a more comprehensive concept of personhood that includes those with acute physical and/or mental dependency that 'cannot be masked'. She also calls for justice for caregivers, including status and remuneration that recognize the moral and interpersonal value of such work and stop measuring its worth primarily in terms of profit, productivity and economic production. Kittay argues that the treatment of caregivers by society and the economy all too often reflects the 'abject' status of those who need such care. In the worst cases, this can be experienced by the carers as implicit permission to abuse and mock helpless and low-status patients simply because they are in an even more 'abject' state than the carers themselves. A cruel exchange of this kind was clearly present in some recent scandals in the English care system involving systematic abuse of acutely autistic, or mentally ill, or 'learning disabled' patients in long-term institutional care (BBC News 2023; Samuel

2023). It is alarmingly unclear how widespread such abuses may be in the British care system.

Relationship in care: women's work?

Everyone who writes about their own experience of giving or receiving care agrees that care intrinsically involves a *relationship* between carer and cared-for, and that this relationship entails reciprocity, just as the parent–child relationship does. Madeleine Bunting concludes at the end of her investigation of care and the current crisis in its provision: 'The deeper cause of the crisis is a fundamental failure to value – and appropriately reward – the centrality of relationship in all care' (Bunting 2020, p 251).

The 'invisible' unpaid care that most women in all classes carry out in the 'private sphere' fundamentally rests on that assumption of 'relationship' that, along with the other assumptions persistently embedded in the female gender role, acts as an unspoken justification of the way the work of care falls so heavily on women: the ideal for males remains a high level of independence and individualism, while for women it assumes interdependence, just as Carol Gilligan argues (Gilligan 1982, 2023). Women who work in demanding jobs find themselves, as I certainly did, pulled in two by this dual commitment to independence and to all the interdependences premised on networks of relationship. Emily Kenway shows just how much it costs a 'responsible relative' to give the invisible care that is assumed to be their (her) duty to a close relative. Yet it is important to consider that according to the 2021 Census for England and Wales, although in every age group up to 75–79 years, females find themselves doing more unpaid caring than men; among the over-eighties, men are more likely than women to find themselves unpaid carers (Office for National Statistics 2023). The cost to unpaid carers is financial, often meaning that the family carer has to give up or cut down paid employment with little monetary compensation from the state; it is also social, as carers find their own lives narrowed to the requirements of the person they care for, with no opportunity of a social life of their own; and it is personal, as many carers find they have no time or energy even to care for their own bodies, appearance or wellbeing (Kenway 2023). James Butler cites a recent calculation that valued such unpaid caregiving in Britain at some £59.5 billion annually (Butler 2023, p 11). The economist Daniel Susskind claims that in the US, 20 million family carers, two thirds of them older women, give $500 billion of unpaid care to adults; while in the UK 6.5 million carers, who are mostly women, perform up to £100 billion of unpaid care each year (Susskind 2020, p 234).

This pattern of invisible care has its visible, paid, analogue not only in the army of paid domestic cleaners that now do some of what the servant class did a century ago in the homes of the 'better off', but also in the care sector of the economy. Carolyn Steedman points out that in the early years of political economy as a 'science', neither Adam Smith nor Karl Marx regarded what servants did at that time as productive 'work' (their model was the new industrialized labour force) and therefore discounted such service labour in their accounts of capitalist modernity (Steedman 2009, p 355). This left a legacy of assumptions that are still working themselves out in an era when the care sector is part of all developed economies. Oxfam published a research report in July 2023 taking up this point (Parvez 2023). It showed that 65 per cent of women's working hours each week are unpaid (that 'second shift'; Hochschild and Machung 1989) and are not included in measures of economic activity even though they constitute a hidden subsidy to the economy. Globally, nearly half of all adults' working hours are similarly excluded from gross domestic product (GDP) calculations. Hence, the Oxfam report sees the measure of GDP as 'not fit for purpose' (Parvez 2023). The measurement of GDP drives policies that depend on women's unpaid work acting as a shock absorber when welfare services are cut. GDP makes no distinction between harmful and beneficial economic activity, a serious consideration as the world faces a climate and environmental crisis. Nor does it take account of what makes for individual or social wellbeing. Although GDP has almost tripled since 1965, the economic wealth it measures has been unequally distributed and has not solved any of the chronic problems of deprivation and inequality. For these reasons, the Oxfam report calls for the use of a wider range of measures by policy makers in order to capture the whole spectrum of economic activities, citing experimental measures of 'wellbeing' as well as the United Nations proposal for measuring 'gross inclusive income' to take account of time use. A number of comparable proposals are currently coming from several directions. It remains to be seen whether they will be taken up by policy makers, although at the moment there is little sign of that.

In common with most other commentators, Butler comments on the gendered nature of care that has persisted even after the welfare state assumed its modern institutional form after the Second World War, building on piecemeal earlier developments in voluntary organizations, private arrangements and fragmentary state provision. He writes:

> Fifty years on, much more care is carried out as work, for a wage and for profit. Three features remain unchanged, however: the centrality of unpaid care work; its apparent invisibility; and its stubbornly gendered quality. Many of those who write on the subject are women whose work is still marginalised. (Butler 2023, p 12)

Emily Kenway believes that the persistent invisibility of the large army of unpaid carers is a symptom of a distorted perception of human life that ignores the fact that most of us will find ourselves on both sides of the care relationship at different points of our lives. In the prologue of her book, Kenway writes of the pressures on carers, like herself, who care for family members:

> I would think about how absurd it all was. That all of us were miserable and suffocating, and yet the experiences stifling us were an inherent part of human life. As inevitable as the hair growing out of our heads, as the need to breathe or sleep, we can be certain that we'll need to give and receive care in our lives. How could something so natural be making us choke? And what would a society look like that understood care as an inherent part of human life instead of a problem in need of a quick fix? (Kenway 2023, p 11)

In our medically sophisticated and demographically ageing societies, governments need to grasp the fact that our care 'crisis' is part of an ongoing and ever-growing *inevitability* rather than something that could be made to disappear with the right policies. Like the poor, care is ever with us. The challenge is to accept that and find ways of providing just and appropriate systems of care that do not crush the carers on whom they depend, who are still predominantly women. Kenway concludes with a warning to her readers about the need to confront squarely that we as individuals as well as our politicians are inured to looking away from reality. She writes:

> The real care crisis is within and between each of us, because together we create a society that side-steps the brute truth about human frailty, and therefore fails to create the systems and structures we need … . For me, this re-education about mortality has been the greatest lesson and the most brutal gift about being a caregiver. (Kenway 2023, pp 287, 289)

The period since the Second World War has seen a revolution in women's employment, as we have had occasion to note. The demographic game-changers underlying that have been smaller families, greater longevity and increases in social and geographical mobility. Today, very few families in any class contain women who remain entirely outside the paid labour market. Laura Schwartz sees the ubiquity of women's paid employment as the main reason most couples are no longer able to do for themselves all the ordinary domestic labour required by the modern household, even when men are willing to do their fair share; this applies with even more force to care work in the home – childcare, eldercare, care for sick or disabled members of the household or of the wider family network. Hence the emergence of the 'care sector' of the formal economy. This sector is made up of all the services provided by a mixture of state and private organizations, some of them franchised by the state, usually through local authorities, to provide services that the state is now legally bound to supply. This includes the health service – that is, the institutional provision under the aegis of the quasi-sacred but underfunded and overburdened NHS and the welfare system, many of whose functions it is the statutory duty of local authorities to provide, and social care, which is organized through local authorities to provide care in homes and in residential settings to those who cannot live independently without help. Care workers are paid employees. They work in many institutional contexts – children's homes, networks of foster families, residential homes for the disabled, care homes for the elderly, day centres and respite centres – plus there is a whole army of adult social care workers who tend to the sick, elderly or disabled, including people with dementia, in their own homes. An additional network of ancillary professional workers services many of the institutions providing care – these include pharmacists, physiotherapists, paramedics, social workers, psychiatrists, psychologists, counsellors and many others. A running sore in the body of the welfare state is the anomaly of dementia sufferers who are not included under the 'health' category and whose care is therefore not the responsibility of the NHS but of even less well resourced social care. In an ageing population, the incidence of dementia is steadily rising, making this a serious and growing problem. The Alzheimer's Dementia Hub reports that in 2023 there were some 944,000 dementia patients in Britain and around 700,000 unpaid family carers. The number of dementia sufferers is expected to rise steeply, predicted to reach one million by 2030 and two million by 2050, with one in three of us likely to develop the condition in our lifetime (Alzheimer's Dementia Hub 2023). At the moment, dementia care is largely funded and/or directly managed by the family under a means test which requires many dementia sufferers to sell their homes to finance their care, marking them out from their peers whose problem – cancer, Parkinson's disease, motor neurone disease – is unequivocally 'medical' and therefore comes under the NHS rather than the Cinderella service of social care. The Alzheimer's Dementia Hub reports that one in two of the British population will be affected by dementia at some point in their lives, either suffering from the condition or caring for a sufferer. In the words of the title of James Butler's article: 'This concerns everyone' (Butler 2023).

Full-time residential care for the elderly and disabled, including dementia sufferers, is a particular source of political and economic difficulty. Both James Butler and Emma Dowling point to the deeply problematic consequences for the service when it passed from local authority direct provision to private providers to whom the state, via local commissioning authorities, provides large subventions of public finance (Dowling 2022; Butler 2023). The justification for this privatization was that markets make private firms more efficient than direct state provision, which lacks market discipline to check complacency and wasteful practices. These private companies mostly work for profit and currently provide 84 per cent of residential care beds. Both James Butler and Emma Dowling emphasize the negative effects of a system by which large private organizations, notably investment banks and corporate asset management, have bought up residential care homes with borrowed funds and then loaded the debt not onto the purchasing umbrella company but onto the care homes. Individual care homes are often embedded in complex, multilevel corporate structures that mystify the ownership of specific homes or care companies and thus can be used to mask tax avoidance. Many care homes, such as the chain of homes run by Four Seasons which folded in 2016, have been forced to close when they cannot service their debt while still making profits for the ultimate corporate owners. Such failures are all too likely in a system which, in addition, routinely cross-subsidizes state-funded residents by increasing fees to cover the shortfall in state welfare contributions.

Long crisis in the care sector during the 21st century

As early as 1999, the Royal Commission on Long Term Care for the Elderly warned of the need to increase funding for healthcare in a fast-ageing demographic. It was followed by two reports commissioned by The King's Fund: the Wanless report in 2002 on health provision (Wanless 2002) and the Barker report in 2014 on the future of health and social care (Barker 2014). These investigations recommended a radical rethink of services; the Barker report made the integration of health and social care a priority along with substantial increases in funding. The Dilnot report in 2011 found the social care system 'not fit for purpose' and again recommended increased funding and structural reform (Commission on Funding of Care and Support 2011), while two years later, the Cavendish review on healthcare assistants and support workers in the NHS and social care settings, made wide-ranging recommendations to improve training and raise the level of skills and remuneration for these two large sectors of the care workforce (Cavendish 2013).

The important and widely quoted report on social justice and health inequalities, *Fair Society, Healthy Lives*, by Sir Michael Marmot, published in 2010 with a follow-up review ten years on by Professor Marmot and his associates at the Institute of Health Equity, definitively demonstrated the direct relation between health inequalities and other social inequalities (Marmot 2010; Marmot et al 2020). There has even been an Archbishops' Commission on Reimagining Care, which published its report in January 2023, proposing a National Care Covenant involving citizens, families, communities and the state to ensure a new deal for unpaid carers, better remuneration for those working in the care sector and a universal entitlement to social care parallel to the universal entitlement to healthcare under the NHS (Archbishops' Commission on Reimagining Care 2023). Numerous charities and voluntary associations, such as Age UK, continually call for reform of the care system. Yet, despite governments of various stripes accepting the findings and recommendations of successive official reports, no effective action had been taken by the onset of the COVID-19 pandemic in 2020. Verbal assurances from successive prime ministers since the end of the pandemic have done nothing to change that situation; in summer 2024 it still remains to be seen what precisely the new Labour government will do. The reform and integration of health and social care is forever intended but never enacted; it is always 'unaffordable' in the present circumstances.

The current state of social care is a good index of the nature and urgency of the immediate care crisis. In October 2022, the number of care workers in adult social care in England fell to the point where substantial numbers of people were left without any care. Unfilled posts rose 52 per cent in a single year, according to the independent body Skills for Care (Skills for Care 2022). They reported that of 1.79 million posts in the sector, 165,000 were left unfilled, 50,000 more than the previous year, representing a vacancy rate of 10 per cent, with a turnover rate of 29 per cent. Skills for Care predicted that by 2035, some 480,000 new posts would be required on top of the present 1.79 million. The report noted that four out of five comparable jobs pay more than the median wage for carers, 28 per cent of whom are over 55 years old. It is common knowledge that supermarket work pays better and demands less. Nadra Ahmed, Chair of the National Care Association, told the *Financial Times* in January 2024 that adult care workers would realistically need to be paid £18 an hour (*Financial Times* 2024). The Skills for Care report states that the average care worker's hourly pay is £1 less than a newly hired NHS healthcare assistant, while care workers with five years' experience earn only 7p an hour more than new recruits. Almost a quarter of workers have zero-hours contracts, staff with low levels of education and training have a higher turnover rate and men and White people are disproportionately found in senior posts. In adult social care, 82 per cent of staff are women, 23 per cent come from minority ethnic populations, 16 per cent have non-British nationality and 11 per cent arrived in Britain within a year of their recruitment (Skills for Care 2022). In summer 2023, a BBC radio programme reported evidence of care workers being trafficked from abroad as incidences of modern slavery (File on Four 2023).

The NHS is not much better placed. It too is experiencing a staffing crisis, exacerbated by Britain's exit from the European Union and the arrangement for the free movement of labour, which had provided a significant section of the workforce of both the NHS and social care. The NHS has an enormous backlog of patients waiting for planned procedures, which is currently growing by a million a year and had reached 7.7 million by autumn 2023 (British Medical Association 2024). The problem is made worse by the difficulty of finding hospital beds even for emergency admissions because one in seven patients who are fit for discharge cannot be sent 'home' because of the lack of social care provision: even before the COVID-19 pandemic, hospitals were 'running hot' through the routine practice of maximizing, rather than optimizing, bed occupancy to avoid carrying 'empty beds' (House of Commons Library 2023). Britain's dependence on medical professionals from other countries, particularly from its old colonial territories, is long-standing, as is the country's failure to train sufficient doctors and nurses from among its own nationals.

The staffing shortage has been made worse by the exhaustion of the workforce through the long period of stressful overwork during the pandemic and the consequent deterioration of working conditions, to be followed, once the pandemic ended, by the vast backlog of waiting lists for postponed elective surgery and by the continuous depression of pay in all kinds of care and health work in the decade since the financial crash of 2008 and post-pandemic cost-of-living shocks. All of this has led to a persistent stream of trained and experienced staff leaving for better pay and conditions in other countries or retiring early. This is the backdrop to the spring and summer of rolling strikes by healthcare workers from cleaners to hospital consultants in 2023. NHS England in June 2023 published its long-awaited Workforce Plan for the NHS (NHS England 2023). This promised a doubling of medical school places, 22 per cent of training for clinical staff via new apprenticeship routes, an increase in GP training places by 50 per cent and a near doubling of adult nursing training places by 2031–32. (NHS Long Term Workforce Plan 2023). The Institute for Fiscal Studies responded with an analysis of the implications of the plan (Institute for Fiscal Studies 2023). It calculated that by 2036–37 almost half of all public service employment will be in the NHS and that whereas in 2021–22 the NHS employed 1 in 17 of all workers in England, by 2036–37 this will have risen to 1 in 11 – that is, 9 per cent of all those active in the paid labour market in England. It also warned that the sums that this would require are considerably more than those projected in the Plan, which do not take account of the ongoing increases in the wage bill consequent on the proposed increases in the labour force or the extra equipment that it will require. The Plan's proposed funding in any case assumes a yearly productivity increase of 1.5 per cent to 2 per cent, which is premised partly on increased use of technology. Such a potential underfunding of the service's real minimal requirements will fall short of solving the stressful working conditions that are driving doctors to find work in other countries, or of securely reducing the long waiting lists for elective surgery and the pressures on emergency departments.

In addition, there is a severe crisis in the availability of NHS dental services alongside the expansion of private dentists, which remain unaffordable for the low-paid, resulting in swathes of the retired and the low-paid going without dental care for years, even decades. Most commentaries argue that the root problem is the systematic underfunding of NHS dental services and the unsatisfactory contracts for NHS dentists. Recently, there have been fears that ophthalmology, notably in relation to cataract surgery, is developing a parallel problem.

There is no mystery, then, about the nature of the care and health crises; both have been extensively analysed and government has a considerable library of reports on which to draw. The effects on the need for health and social care among an ageing population has been understood and widely discussed for some decades – about 20 per cent of the British population is currently over 65 and this share is growing steadily, with the fastest-rising age group being my own, the over 85s. In July 2023 the Health Foundation issued the *Health in 2040* report, which predicts 9.1 million people in 2040 living with major illness, an increase of 2.5 million on the 2019 figure (Health Foundation 2023). Much of this illness is likely to be made up of anxiety, depression, chronic pain and diabetes, conditions that will require more general practice services. While there is likely to be an increase of over one third in the numbers living with major illnesses, this will have to be financed by the taxes of a working population that will have grown by only 4 per cent. The Institute for Fiscal Studies response to the NHS Plan for its workforce calculates that the (probably underestimated) level of funding promised in the Plan will mean a 3.6 per cent increase in health funding and amount to 2 per cent more of GDP (Institute for Fiscal Studies 2023).

The two widely praised reports on health inequalities by epidemiologist Michael Marmot provide the background against which these cost figures should be seen. The Marmot reports have been widely endorsed – indeed, Professor Sir Michael Marmot was made a Companion of Honour in the 2023 New Year's Honours List for his services to public health – but no government has yet acted on the central findings and recommendations of his two reports, which, at bottom, constitute a politically embarrassing reminder of the health consequences of the whole range of rising economic and social inequalities which, anyway, cannot in themselves be solved solely by increasing NHS funding. Marmot incontrovertibly demonstrates a systematic relation between health inequalities and other indices of inequality – infant mortality, life expectancy, substandard housing conditions, poverty, including food poverty, insecure or poorly paid work or harmful working conditions, poor education outcomes and disadvantaged communities.

As noted in the review ten years after the original report, '[h]ealth is closely connected with the conditions in which people are born, grow up, live, work and age' (Marmot et al 2020, p 1). It is particularly striking that since the original report in 2010, life expectancy has plateaued (after decades of steadily rising) for all but the most privileged class and the number of years of life spent in poor health has risen, while for women and ethnic minorities in the most disadvantaged communities, life expectancy has actually fallen. Marmot argues, cogently, that interventions that only target the most disadvantaged will make little overall difference to the pattern because disadvantage is systematically graduated; helping only those at the very bottom will leave the next levels above still at multiple systematic disadvantage. Marmot argued in his original report that rather than merely focusing on treating ill health, the perspective should be reversed: 'Well-being should be a more important societal goal than *simply more economic growth*' (Marmot et al 2020, p 1, emphasis added). Marmot recommends community-based initiatives rather than targeting policy on individual- or family-based medical action when illness has already occurred. He advocates a concentration on prevention rather than only crisis intervention. This, of course, rather than simply making the population healthier and reducing the costs to the state, means an increase in survival rates which may well subsequently swell the numbers living with illnesses. Marmot's term for sustainable and equitable action to remedy the problems of health inequality is 'proportionate universalism'. The same holistic logic clearly also applies to social care.

Evidence to the UK COVID-19 Inquiry presented jointly by Sir Michael Marmot and Professor Clare Bambra on 16 June 2023 argued that, in preparing their response to the pandemic, the government already had abundant evidence of the depleted condition of public services and of increasing health inequalities, including the reduction of life expectancy among poor women (Marmot and Bambra 2023). According to their evidence, the disproportionate impact of the COVID-19 infection on people from ethnic minority groups, people who are disabled and members of disadvantaged communities could have been anticipated and addressed. In the event, existing health inequalities caused mortality and morbidity among these sections of the population to be particularly high. In the early weeks of the inquiry in 2023, health experts and even Conservative politician Oliver Letwin, who had had responsibility for pandemic planning under David Cameron's coalition government, admitted the authorities were woefully unprepared and the health system lacked resilience, though Cameron and George Osborne defended their policies of austerity as economically necessary. The inquiry is still ongoing in July 2024.

As we have seen, the roots of the care crisis are many. Although simply spending more money is not in itself a solution to fixing a complex system, it is a myth that more money will not improve outcomes in the care sector. Britain is no better than average in the league tables of European and other developed societies both in its per capita expenditure on the health and care sector and in its health outcomes; increasing the per capita inputs *will* improve outcomes. To solve the current crisis in the NHS, and even more so in social care, the government will need to spend considerably more money on infrastructure, training and remuneration of health and care workers; restructure provisions to focus more on prevention and on community action, which will involve addressing inequalities in all areas, including housing, education and work; and rethink its assumptions about health and care always being more efficiently delivered through 'markets'. If Britain is to build civilized 21st-century provision of welfare and nurture a harmonious civic life that no longer leads to multiple penalization of those at the bottom of its pyramid of inequalities, government will first have to find money and resources for the health and social care sector. The two sectors are interdependent, and without a solution for social care, no amount of increased funding for the NHS will clear the backlog of hospital waiting lists or make hospitals less stressful workplaces for health workers. The Secretary of State for Health and Social Care in the 2024 Labour administration, Wes Streeting, has promised a two-term plan to clear the backlog, but only time will tell whether he can succeed. Although solving all these problems for good looks politically implausible, fortunately, the threat to the preservation of the welfare state is currently exercising political imaginations in some unexpected places, a subject to which I now turn.

8

Rethinking Capitalism, the Future of Work and the Role of Care

Critics of capitalism: Thomas Piketty

The prolonged crisis in the care sector predates the 2007–08 financial upheaval but has grown worse in the era of austerity that followed. Many observers, including Sir Michael Marmot, judge the clear correlation between government policies of austerity and the increase in health inequalities as almost certainly causal: the near-collapse of social care as government imposed swingeing cuts in welfare funding as the price of rescuing the banks is indicative. The crisis in health and social care is part of the collateral damage of the financial crisis and the intensification of inequalities that it revealed. One of the most influential critiques of the situation came not from investigations in the health and care sector, but from an economist. In 2013 the book by French economist Thomas Piketty, *Capital in the Twenty-First Century*, became an unexpectedly influential bestseller; it had sold 2.4 million copies by 2016. (Piketty 2013). Piketty spells out the way inequality in developed capitalist societies has been rising since around 1980, reverting to the original pattern of high inequalities that characterized industrial capitalism from its infancy and has now recurred after a period of redistribution after the Second World War. Piketty sees the financial crisis of 2007–08 as the system again working normally by prioritizing capital over income, rather than being simply the temporary consequence of inadequate financial controls or bad monetary and fiscal policies in the immediate past. Using a battery of historical data starting from the beginning of the Industrial Revolution, Piketty demonstrates that, with the exception of the long mid-20th-century Keynesian era after the Second World War, extreme inequality had been the norm in industrial capitalism everywhere it took root, and became so again after 1980. Since that point, income and wealth have been steadily redistributed to a very narrow elite – Piketty calls it 'the top 1%'. The financial crisis of 2008 exposed this and illustrates capitalism's reversion to type after the exceptional postwar period of high, redistributive tax policy, which came to a juddering end in the 1980s with the emergence of what became known as neoliberalism.

Piketty challenges economists with his innovative method and argument. His numerous graphs showing the pattern of inequalities over time and across the developed world are meticulously grounded in hard historical data, and his method of measuring the return on capital relative to growth is difficult for economists of any school to dismiss as heretical. Piketty's case is that where the rate of return on capital outstrips the rate of economic growth, capital/wealth systematically outstrips income. Slow economic growth allied with better financial return results in the increasing inequalities that have become ingrained once more in the system after a period in which the overall rising level of growth benefited enough people outside the privileged elite to deflect attention from relative inequalities. The financial crisis made those inequalities and the direction of travel clearly visible once more.

Piketty argues that exceptional conditions made possible the construction of the welfare state after the Second World War by enhancing the power of the state to raise taxation; these were: total war and continuing threats of war; the postwar need to rebuild war-damaged economies and social infrastructure; the power of organized labour in the heavily industrialized economies of the period; and demographic and technological change. These conditions coincided after the Second World War to boost the legitimacy of the state's tax-raising activity along democratic lines that redistributed wealth and income downwards and funded a 'welfare state' that benefited all citizens. Conditions have changed since then. The 1980s saw the establishment of the Thatcher–Reagan era, bringing in neoliberalism. Piketty believes that in this recent phase of capitalism, inequalities of wealth have been given more legitimacy because the most privileged strata have spread wealth to the managerial class in a way that 19th-century industrialism failed to do. Nevertheless, the privileged elite that benefits most from capital accumulation is continuous from past to present but is now internally divided between what Piketty calls the 'Brahmin left' (with cultural and social as well economic capital) and the 'Merchant right' (a business class, including a new group of 'plutocrats'). While Marx defined the key variable as *production* – its structures, ownership and control – in contemporary capitalism the key variable, and therefore the key problem, has become *distribution* of wealth. As wealth becomes ever more concentrated in 'the top 1%', the only way to redress the imbalance is through highly redistributive tax policies, as it was after the Second World War.

In later work with various collaborators, Piketty has somewhat modulated his argument (Alvaredo et al 2018). The prime exemplar of his model of capitalism's tendency to revert to high levels of inequality is the US, and

European societies have shown some resistance to US extremes. Continued commitment to (relatively) high levels of taxation and a redistributive welfare state has made Europe the outlier in the global capitalist pattern of increasingly wide income and wealth inequalities (Desmond 2023). For Piketty and his followers, the ability of the state to intervene in capitalist distribution of wealth and income is key to the continuation of effective welfare states. Finding adequate political and moral legitimation to support redistributive policies against the self-interest of the most privileged and influential elites is the key to tackling the care crisis, and is no easy task.

Associated revisions: Mike Savage

Piketty has not been a lone voice: many social scientists have joined the debate. Indeed, social scientists researching social policy have a long tradition of criticizing the effects of the 'free market' on the delivery and effectiveness of welfare. It is a truism of such analyses that, despite fears and claims that much welfare spending goes to the 'undeserving', who cheat the system, all the evidence is that the middle classes gain most from welfare systems, including healthcare. One indicative example of this kind of research is a sharp critique of neoliberalism in British pension provision published in 2015 by the social historian John Macnicol (Macnicol 2015).

Postcolonial theorists such as Talal Asad have laid the foundation for a critique of the global consequences of contemporary capitalism. Other contributions to the critique come from what might seem an unexpected direction, the sociology and anthropology of religion, including critical studies of Pentecostalism as a cultural manifestation of neoliberalism's global reach as well as a prophylactic against the worst of its effects, particularly on poor and Indigenous peoples (Robbins 2004). Mathew Guest provides a wide-ranging and perceptive analysis of the way neoliberalism has infiltrated what is taken for granted in cultures dominated by neoliberal economics, including religions and the intellectual analyses of them, as well as the political assumptions states make about religious groups (Guest 2022, especially pp 85–108). He argues that the cultural mutations of neoliberalism have delegitimated the role of ethical judgements in many fields, including universities and the academic disciplines and the research they host, because 'neoliberalism is not simply a dimension of contemporary life but an ideology that shapes the way in which people think' (Guest 2022, p 167). Economic cost–benefit calculations routinely trump ethical judgements. As we shall see later, some prominent economists and financial technocrats share his judgement that separating morals from markets is a mistake with extensive and deleterious consequences for society.

A significant contribution to the debate stimulated by Piketty is the work of British political sociologist Mike Savage. Following Piketty's work, Savage revisited the analysis of social class in *The Return of Inequality: Social Change and the Weight of the Past* (Savage 2021). Savage begins from Piketty's analysis but modulates it with arguments about the ongoing legacy of empire, showing, for instance, that four 'increasingly powerful imperial blocs' – the US and its Anglophone satellites (Australia, Canada and the UK), China, India and Russia – between them account for half the global super-rich, the US especially (Savage 2021, p 166). Yet he also shows that members of the global top 10 per cent of the income scale are currently less likely to be found in European societies than in Asia, because many European states have limited the growth of income inequality through commitment to 'higher taxation and a redistributive welfare state' (Savage 2021, p 144). In 1980, Europe was considerably more unequal than China, India and Russia and only a little less unequal than the US, whereas today Europe is the outlier, a relatively less unequal region in a world of increasingly wide inequalities. Savage, like Piketty, identifies a group of European nations as 'countervailing exemplars to the dystopian American model' (Savage 2021, p 144). Even so, he sees serious challenges to democratic political systems in the new phase of rising inequality as the processes of capitalist accumulation disproportionately enrich a small, highly privileged elite, linked globally in transnational networks of privilege and wielding an apparent stranglehold on political processes of distribution of wealth and income. Britain's position straddling the less unequal countries of Western Europe and the particularly unequal capitalism of the US has been underlined by Britain's exit from the European Union.

Savage's main thesis concerns the persistent weight of past history, a position with which I am sympathetic, especially since part of my argument parallels his, turning on just how much has *not* changed in women's lives, notably the continuities in their 'reproductive labour' and caring roles even after entering the labour market en masse. Mike Savage is highly critical of the dominance of what he terms 'modernist' models that make sharp divisions between past, present and future (a relic of 19th-century models of progressive 'evolutionary stages'), and he is unpersuaded that modernity transcends historical specificities. Those 'modernist' innovations that are meant to guarantee the openness of present and future – such as transparency, meritocratic education systems, the erosion of the kudos of old elite cultural tastes in favour of more democratized cultural styles – on closer inspection turn out to conceal the persistence, indeed the consolidation, of the privileges of the elites who had benefited most from earlier capital accumulation. This is true even as they admit a trickle of new members in successive generations and as the style in which privilege is culturally signalled alters (what indicates 'cultural capital'). The legacy of the past lies in the historically generated categories built into systems of understanding and the representation of social divisions.

In the wake of empire in the 19th and 20th centuries, nation states constructed the political fields in which power was exercised and contested. These national political fields slowly admitted categories – initially only the men – that had been marginalized and excluded. Savage argues that the classic 'categorical identities' – class, race, gender – were the products of an 'incessant boundary marking' associated with Imperial capitalist projects around the globe in the 19th century. They marked the trusted insider from the untrustworthy outsider (including the distinction between 'good' and 'disreputable' women). These exclusionary definitions and boundaries prompted outsiders within the nation state to struggle for access to citizenship rights and acceptance in a way that ultimately shaped the political sphere and its democratic institutions. Savage believes the conditions of today's new inequalities have begun to unravel these arrangements, among other things by making it clear that inequalities are not simply historical residues that will automatically fade away but are the consequence of entrenched processes related to the nature and history of capitalism.

One element in the radical reconfiguration of national political fields that Savage identifies is the measurement of relative differences, introduced by the social sciences in the 20th century, that has largely turned 'class' from something once experienced as an ontological, natural division into a probabilistic category produced by relativities of rights and life chances. In the currently shifting 'field dynamics' of national politics, social class is no longer the obvious correlate or predictor of electoral behaviour; democratic authority to control and rein in capitalist accumulation and its attendant power is under strain; and there is no certainty that European states will be capable of supporting redistributive welfare policies indefinitely. Yet, although class may have lost its former tight connection with electoral choice as political parties have splintered and changed, it nevertheless remains a good predictor of the *level* of political engagement: the privileged engage in the public sphere far more, and far more confidently, than the underprivileged, who feel excluded and discounted. All this echoes much of what we saw in the discussion of Britain's post-Brexit 'new tribes', including the way the educationally mobile join Piketty's Brahmin left while the left behind White working class tacks itself onto the Merchant right, and attitudes to race and immigration act as the litmus test dividing liberal from conservative identities. Savage points out that the Blair government 'recast Labour as a party oriented towards a middle-class electorate' and that after it lost power and moved to the Left, the Party did not lose this character (Savage 2021, p 301). The general election of 2019 was the first time that more of the working-class electorate voted for the (Boris Johnson) Conservatives than for Labour. (The election of 2024 tested this contingent switch without definitively reversing it.)

Savage points to an inversion of the historical Left/Right dichotomy in the 21st century as the 'progressive left' has found itself increasingly defending what he calls 'older modalities of public provision', such as in health and social care, against the assault of a neoliberal phalanx on the 'right', intent on speeding up economic innovation and capital accumulation through policies of deregulation and rejecting tradition; political attitudes to the British NHS illustrate this very clearly. This shift of political alignment is another element sufficiently disruptive to the 'field dynamics' of national politics and the traditional class association of political parties to open a fissure into which 'identity' or 'lifestyle' politics could slip and trump material concerns.

Savage's view of the displacement of class as a potent political category adds an additional twist to analyses of the rise of identity politics which was discussed in Chapter 3, particularly with reference to the arguments of Kenan Malik. Savage uses the term 'visceral' to characterize the self-identities that are largely written on the body – sex, gender, race. Visceral divisions resist absorption into the probabilistic categories of relative rights and social opportunities that have played a part in unravelling the electoral salience of class. Visceral identities refuse to play by the old 'rules of the game' laid down in earlier political contestation among rival elites and between elites and excluded groups. This refusal disrupts established practices and expectations. Moreover, just as at the height of empire, the top elites today are still overwhelmingly made up of White men. Exclusion by gender and race is a legacy of the Imperial era when, as categories, women and 'other races' were ontologically barred from participation in power. Consequently, the identity politics of these excluded categories copy the radicalism that marked the struggles of excluded and marginalized peoples in Europe's Imperial territories during their campaigns for dignity and national independence. Savage regards the uncompromising stance of identity politics as a way the still marginalized reject the categories imposed on them 'from above', including material (class) ones, and instead prioritize chosen, visceral, self-definition. Their struggle is about recognition and is often driven by rage at a long past of exclusion and exploitation.

What Savage calls 'the capture of elites by plutocrats' in the latest rise in capitalist inequalities, and the populist wave of electoral politics across the globe that it has fed, have further destabilized 'nation spaces' as the political field of action and have disrupted established democratic processes. This is illustrated by the careers of self-made plutocrat politicians, such as Donald Trump and Jair Bolsonaro, who use an anti-establishment rhetoric to appeal to a blue-collar electorate. Despite his pessimistic diagnosis, Savage concludes his book with a plea for an end to the 'growth paradigm' that has for so long dominated economic and political thinking, ignoring the way poorer and less economically developed societies bear so much of its cost, and with a call to address the urgent problem of climate change. He believes democratic societies must find ways of holding capitalism's winners to account and of enhancing the role of public stewardship. This should encompass 'richer conceptions of human life and the human condition' beyond those of the market. To do all this would be, finally, to address and redress capitalism's inequalities. Such a programme is more easily rhetorically urged than politically achieved. Like Savage, I have to leave the 'how' hanging for the moment.

Radical critiques of *Homo economicus*: straws in the wind or signs of change?

Other economic critiques have rounded out arguments about the weakening of the ability of democratic politics to hold capitalism to account. Among others, Quinn Slobodian, Brett Christophers, and Kojo Koram have drawn attention to the way the global actors in today's financialized capitalism, notably libertarian ideologues, investors and asset managers, have contrived to construct 'zones' and 'territories' (freeports, offshore tax havens, postcolonial neoliberal outposts) and techniques of 'asset management' by which the priorities of commerce and profit cannot be restrained by the demands of citizens for 'welfarism' or democratic control (Christophers 2023; Koram 2023; Slobodian 2023). Kojo Koram points out that the state does not wither away in the face of such developments but, rather, finds itself recruited to 'de-risk the project of investing in a particular jurisdiction by socialising any losses' (Koram 2023, p 12). He cites the use of British Overseas Territories for such projects. Other analysts of the history of empire have similarly been struck, as Mike Savage is, by the effect on the home nation of the end of empire, contributing to an erosion of the national project and its democratic processes (Kumar 2021; Koram 2022; Ward 2023).

In his discussion of Christophers' analysis of 'asset management', Koram stresses that the practice occurs at a considerable distance from any actual production of goods and services, not least because much of the profit made by asset managers is in fees that are paid long before it can definitively be established whether or not the assets have been well managed. Christophers describes the 1980s and the period after the debt crisis of 2007–08 as pivotal times in the development of a shadow structure of asset management. Money gathered from individual citizens in small regular sums through pension schemes, insurance companies and the like are invested by asset managers, not primarily into financial assets but into the infrastructure on which we all depend – housing, schools, bridges, farms, care homes, gas pipes, water pipes, reservoirs, rail tracks, wind farms, parking lots, toll roads – 'the physical as well as financial world around us' (Christophers 2023, p 8). In many ways, Christophers' argument is a more radical extension of what came to be known as 'the Titmuss paradigm', after Richard Titmuss' analysis of the interconnection of private and state investment in pension and insurance schemes in the postwar British welfare state (Stewart 2020). Since the 1980s, much of the control of such assets has passed into the hands of 'private equity' of the kind that we noted in Chapter 7 buying up and leveraging debt onto care home companies like Four Seasons. The process has been intensified since the debt crisis resulted in the increased regulation of banks. This increased regulation strengthened the incentive for asset management to use 'private' property transactions that are less constrained by the need for public disclosure than is 'public equity'. By these means, Christophers argues, the profits on funds invested by the many are redirected to the elite, Piketty's 'top 1%' (Christophers 2023). Laleh Khalili sums up Christophers' picture of these innovations as 'the mechanisms through which private equity firms and asset managers have devoured the public infrastructure on which our lives depend, in service of private profit' (Khalili 2023, p 21). Part of the story is the way the privatized water companies in England (by contrast with the publicly owned water companies in the European Union) have underinvested in infrastructure, paid excessive profits to shareholders and inflated executive salaries, all financed by debt. They regularly discharge untreated sewage into rivers and onto beaches in the 2020s in spite of the existence of regulatory institutions that are meant to hold them to account. This ongoing scandal has so far (as of summer 2024) led to the (forced) resignation of the CEO of Thames Water and an ongoing attempt to strengthen regulation and prevent the companies from introducing large increases to customer bills to make up for their long failure to invest in infrastructure. In 2024, it seems difficult for the Labour government to prevent the companies' enormous debts from being transferred to the public purse or directly to the customers.

The political economist William Davies points out that the use of private asset management by the state itself is a continuing element in the funding of health and social care (a system larger and more difficult to manage than any modern private company) as well as in the development of the 'green economy' as governments attempt to reach 'zero carbon' by 2050, as all the main British political parties have promised. Davies sees 'a new vogue for industrial policy' in contemporary states, including the European Union and the US, as a way to protect national economic security when globalization is visibly breaking down under the disruptions of recent hot and cold wars and the search for a green transition. He notes that there has been considerable criticism of public money being channelled to private firms 'in the form of tax credits and subsidies – a policy aimed at getting large asset managers on board' (Davies 2023, p 9). He claims '[f]und managers are being offered a huge fiscal carrot, and risking little regulatory stick', adding that such policies were almost certainly abused during the pandemic in the procurement process (Davies 2023, p 9). Davies' overall message is that most Western analysts now agree that the state must play a big role in managing the economy, despite the trust many politicians and technocrats appear to have in the neoliberal dogma that markets are the best allocators of resources and that government hand-outs only delay necessary adjustments. He believes the demands of citizens for government assistance have become the norm not the exception – in the fiscal crisis of 2007–08, in the pandemic of 2020–23, in the cost-of-living crisis and in the drive for a green transition. Davies also cites the finding of the International Monetary Fund that the level of profits made a larger contribution to rising prices than wage levels in the Eurozone over the past two years of inflation. (Compare the British government's insistence on exactly the opposite during the wave of rail strikes and strikes in the health sector in 2023 and 2024, towards the end of Sunak's tenure as prime minister). The point was reiterated by Egyptian American economist Mohammed El-Erian and Italian American English economist Mariana Mazzucato in a discussion on the BBC's *Newsnight* in November 2023, when they jointly insisted that cutting taxes in Britain in recent decades has only boosted profits for private wealth without increasing investment for growth, such as for infrastructure, new green industries or counteracting climate change (El-Erian and Mazzuccato 2023). Davies contends that the new paradigm of the 'active state' in contemporary political economy is unlikely to unravel the economic status quo but will continue to embed the role of private finance and asset management ever more centrally in welfare provision while modifying 'economics as usual' only at the edges.

Kojo Koram concludes his argument about the distortions built into asset management and 'free zones' by contemporary capitalism as follows: 'The point of carving out these gaps in public authority is to fix the market, not to free it; to gamify the economy so that a return on investment is guaranteed whether the investor performs well or not' (Koram 2023, p 12). This is surely one of the drivers of Piketty's conclusion about increasing inequalities as the return on capital exceeds the rise in incomes. In these conditions, what hope is there for Mike Savage's better public stewardship, a richer conception of human life, sustainable nationalisms and a real attempt to control man-made climate change? Or for a long-term solution to the care crisis?

Ethical failure or structural dysfunction? A view from cybernetics

Critiques of the kind just outlined have been amplified in an accessible ergonomic guide to our current managerial, political and economic woes, *The Unaccountability Machine*, by Daniel Davies, an economist, ergonomic theorist and former investment banker (Davies 2024). Davies argues that over the last century an industrialized structure of decision-making has emerged by which important institutions are run by systems operating according to standardized sets of information and rules of procedure rather than on individual human judgements and direct evidence. An almost inevitable system dysfunction rather than deliberate conspiracy or corruption is the root cause of what he calls today's 'polycrises' in economic and political institutions, including the health and social welfare systems.

Davies sets out the ergonomic model of any managerial system as a flow of communication between different levels of management and responsibility. Each level holds a 'black box' of data and communication, which if reviewed in total would overwhelm any one human intelligence, but when split into sections can be handled by standardized processes at each management level. This works, provided everyone follows the rulebook rather than using individual judgement when anomalies and challenges arise.

This structure necessarily creates what he calls 'accountability sinks' in all complex institutions, from industrial firms to government administrations, banks, insurance companies or universities. If everyone is following the rules of a standardized system at the appropriate level, no one individual has the responsibility to open the black box to check the continuing relevance and accuracy of the information on which the rules were based in the first place, or of the data condensed into the standardized information exchanged, which nowadays may often take the form of a computer algorithm. Systems of this kind have to treat the rulebook as the ultimate authority against which no appeal is allowed. In this way, the smooth 'mechanical' operation of the system can be assured, saved from frequent disruption through appeals and litigation.

The responsibility for tweaking the rules or scrutinizing the continuing accuracy and relevance of the data in the communication flow lies at particular levels of the system whose function is to take in information and act on it. If these levels atrophy, are bypassed or fail to get the relevant information in time, the system will become dysfunctional and those whose lives are affected by its decisions experience accountability shortfall, failure or, at worst, a crisis of legitimacy. Thus, accountability sinks are necessary but can also cause serious trouble. This is exactly what Davies believes has occurred. In particular, he cites the decimation of swathes of middle management through which communication flows; the outsourcing of subsections of the organization's operations, which creates new boundaries between the organization and the outside environment; and the failure of top management levels to understand their function of monitoring the purpose of the institution. Lost levels of middle management mean the two-way flow of communication within the organization develops blind spots; new boundaries with the outside environment make it harder to get relevant information to the organizational level that needs to react to it; and the failure at the top means that information from outside the organization, including from the population affected by the organization's decisions, may not be heard and addressed. Davies terms this failure at the top the 'decrebration' of the system – the atrophy of what the pioneer management theorist Stafford Beer (the hero of Davies' book) called 'the brain of the firm' (Davies 2024, p 105). Davies summarizes, 'a given system has the potential to achieve stability only if every source of variability from the environment is matched by an equal or greater source of variety in the regulatory system' (Davies 2024, p 105). This is 'Ashby's principle of sufficient variety'. The actions and adjustments this requires can be almost continuous as both environment and organization change. This is why Davies believes all institutions need the equivalent of a red warning light or emergency lever to indicate distress or danger when the system is malfunctioning because it is not adjusting to vital information from the environment.[1]

Davies sees the 2007–08 financial crisis and the export of the 'market' model from economic institutions into other parts of the social system, notably the political system and public service organizations, as the root of these polycrises. He also emphasizes the importance of revisiting, from time to time, the human judgement used in the choice of criteria for standardizing information, which may contain unrecognized biases and prejudices carried over from earlier assumptions. However far information is condensed and processes standardized, at bottom, their usefulness depends on the human criteria that govern the selection of the data.

In addition, Davies attributes much of the 'blame' for recent widespread institutional malfunction to the neoliberal economic orthodoxy that followed the theories of Milton Friedman in the 1970s. In the 1980s, from being a theoretical discipline modelling economic systems, economics morphed into an ideology that believed first that it was describing reality and then that this model was a prescription. 'The market' came to be treated as a superhuman intelligence and 'Friedmanism' decreed that the supreme goal and purpose of organizations was to make profits, overriding all other rationales, including providing a service, making useful goods, running a health or care system for the benefit of recipients or taking account of the likely future. Friedman's mantra that the purpose of a firm was to 'maximize shareholder value' became economic orthodoxy. This partly accounts for the decerebration that occurs when 'the brain of the firm' ceases to relate the stated or ostensible purpose of the firm to the outcomes the firm actually achieves. Davies illustrates: 'The only reason we might think that the purpose of an oil company is to destroy life on planet earth is POSIWID – that's what it does!' (Davies 2024, p 267). The Purpose of a System Is What It Does! Not passing on the experience of the complaints department or a spate of negative publicity in the press because the managerial level that once had that duty has been cut out can mean that vital information does not get to the higher level that should address it. Davies continues: 'Every decision-making system set up as a maximizer needs to have a higher-level system watching over it' (Davies 2024, p 270)

One example of the danger of mistaking models for reality in economic thinking that Davies cites is the common acceptance of 2 per cent as the magic limit to the rate of inflation that governments should install in their economic policies, even though that figure was arbitrary. Another consequence that affected welfare services and government administration, where making literal 'profits' did not apply, was to cut down outgoings, the costs on the balance sheet. This led to repeated attempts to do more with less – fewer staff, less expenditure, economies in the cost of infrastructure or reduction of benefits to recipients. Rather than increases in efficiency, this imposition of an inappropriate 'market' model has tended to reduce the quality of public services of all kinds.

The installation of 'profit maximization' as the sacred goal of a complex institution, whatever it had been set up to do, make or perform, had far-reaching consequences which underlay the 2007–08 financial crisis. 'Financialization' saw big organizations develop their own financial arms, and the practice of leveraged debt buyouts became routine. Once the easy pickings had been taken, more dubious purchases were made in order to generate quick profits by swift resales that simply passed debt down the pecking order of organizations. We observed Brett Christophers demonstrating how such practices led to the collapse of private care companies that could not sustain the debt loaded onto them by the purchasing institution. The results of these pyramids of debt could be ignored while they only threatened organizations low in the chain, so long as profits continued to fatten the 'bottom line' of big companies and financial institutions at the top of the chain. The increasing prevalence of debt, which should have acted as a danger signal to the system, was used as a profit maximizer for the big boys of business or sometimes as what Davies calls a 'control system' to discipline managers – for example, those in dependent supply companies – by curbing managerial salaries or the distribution of share options and bonuses to management rather than increasing shareholder dividends. All that fell apart with the collapse of Lehman Brothers, ushering in the financial crisis.

Complex organizations have failed to recognize that stripping out the apparent 'dead wood' in layers of management left the flow of information within the organization and between it and the surrounding environment dangerously deficient. Davies sees the increasing use of consultants for short-term projects as a makeshift reaction to decerebration at the top. He also regards the waves of political populism all over the world as a cry of distress from populations protesting that their institutions and governments are damaging lives – the equivalent of the danger signal or emergency brake that institutions have failed to install. Davies believes we are urgently in need of more appropriate economic models and concludes that we must reform the operation of private equity and, above all, develop new models of corporate governance.

More disquiet among capitalism's technocrats

Davies was for some years a financial technocrat, observing financialized capitalism from the Bank of England. Others were also disturbed by what they saw. In December 2020, the Reith Lectures were given by Mark Carney, the outgoing Governor of the Bank of England (a position he held since 2013), who previously served as Governor of the Bank of Canada (between 2008 and 2013). Carney's title was *How We Get What We Value*, and the lectures were a searching critique of the contemporary working of capitalism. In the book that grew out of the lectures, *Value(s): Building a Better World for All*, he summarizes: 'we have been moving from a market economy to a market society. Increasingly, to be valued, an asset or activity has to be in a market; the price of everything is becoming the value of everything' (Carney 2021, p 3). *Value(s)* is tellingly bookended with a parable about wine and grappa, representing humanity and the market, respectively. The parable was told by Pope Francis at a lunch given at the Vatican for policy makers, business people, academics, labour leaders and charity workers, which Carney attended. Pope Francis explained that the job of his guests was not to do the impossible by turning grappa back into wine, but to achieve the eminently desirable by turning the market back into humanity. The anecdote and its prominence in the book suggest that Carney is deeply informed by Catholic social teaching. In his presentation of the history of economic thinking and his analysis of what is going wrong with capitalism and the financial institutions that serve it, he is clear that the market is useful, even indispensable, as a tool but a monster when it usurps society's moral and spiritual values. Carney believes that we are 'approaching the extremes of commodification as commerce expands deep into the personal and civic realms' (Carney 2021, p 124). The argument draws on contemporary critical economic thinkers such as Mariana Mazzucato (see 2019, 2022), though not directly on Piketty. Carney shows the many ways in which 'market fundamentalism' has undermined the social and moral basis on which the market depends. His analysis is part of a liberal perspective, but it rests on an organic model of society that is unmistakably Catholic Christian. He writes:

> In economics, the combination of subjective value and marginalism changed the perceptions of value from the intrinsic characteristics of a good or service to its exchange value. Its price in the market. In the process, the importance of distribution of income and the distinction between productive and unproductive activities were downplayed, and with them, corporate purpose and national ideals were devalued. (Carney 2021, p 124)

The founders of economic thought were never deluded about the need for moral and social values to underpin and control markets. Carney writes:

> Markets are social constructs, whose effectiveness is determined partly by the rules of the state and partly by the values of society. If left unattended they will corrode those values. We must concentrate on rebuilding social capital to make markets work. To do so, individuals and their firms must rediscover their sense of solidarity and responsibility for the system. (Carney 2021, p 12)

He concludes that individuals and firms can do this only by rediscovering a proper humility and sense of responsibility, which will also mean recognizing human interdependence and communal and social purpose. Mark Carney advocates 'a life of moral not market sentiments: a life that seeks to advance the trinity of distributive justice, equality of opportunity and fairness across generations' (Carney 2021, p 522).

Both Mike Savage and Mark Carney end their diagnoses of the problems of contemporary capitalism with invocations of moral sentiments – appeals to cultural and moral change as the only way to address the chronic inequities and distortions of capitalism. Another former international banker, Minouche Shafik, joins them in calling for a reset of contemporary capitalism and its values and institutions. She laments the prevalence of the principle that 'you're on your own', which she sees as toxic for human wellbeing. It results in 'the politics of anger, an epidemic of mental health issues and both young and old fearing for their futures. Yet in many areas bearing risks individually is not just inequitable, it is also far less efficient and productive than sharing them across society' (Shafik 2021, pp 164–5). She places her argument in the 'social contract' tradition, which recognizes our continuing debt to each other as citizens and the utility of providing jointly for our common needs as more efficient as well as more ethically justified than leaving it to the (fictional) atomized modern 'individual' to provide for themself. Shafik directly illustrates Piketty's argument about rising inequalities and the way that economic growth disproportionately benefits a small elite at the expense of the rest. She reviews comparative data in separate chapters on children, education, health, work, old age and generations. Her conclusion is:

> We owe each other more. A more generous and inclusive social contract would recognise our interdependencies, provide minimum protections to all, share some of the risks collectively and ask everyone to contribute as much as they can for as long as they can. This is not about increasing the welfare state, but about investing in people and building a new system of risk sharing to increase overall well-being. (Shafik 2021, p 138)

She adds: 'Change will come inevitably because the forces of technology, demography and environmental pressures will drive it' (Shafik 2021, p 188) May these new 'forces', perhaps, act in the same way the postwar conditions after 1945 made possible the Keynesian revolution and the creation of the welfare settlement?

The Fourth Industrial Revolution: artificial intelligence to the rescue?

It has become common to refer to the latest stage of technological innovation, from the internet and digital communication to the development and application of AI, as the Fourth Industrial Revolution. Everywhere today we see predictions of what it means for politics and the economy, especially for the future of employment, but there is little agreement other than that it is bringing radical change to everyday lives. The political implications of the Fourth Industrial Revolution are interpreted differently by various commentators. Mike Savage sees the digital revolution in communications as yet another re-inscription of privilege into a new modality and a novel range of institutions rather than, as its pioneers often claim, a benign democratization of knowledge. He writes that 'the purported "knowledge economy" actually intensifies the mobilization of past activity, through the hoovering up and manipulation of previously accumulated mountains of data' (Savage 2021, p 251). Existing elites are disproportionately benefited by the profits of the corporations that deploy these mountains of data and by the political leverage that the manipulation and application of such data makes possible. Shoshana Zuboff argues angrily that much of that valuable data – our opinions, likes and dislikes, the subjects of our online searches, purchases and much else – is taken by 'big data' corporations without our permission (Zuboff 2019).

Other commentators see different potentials in contemporary information technology, especially AI, in the context of population change and changes in generational balance. The developed world has a predominance of older generations who dominate the power and wealth structure and consume an increasing proportion of health and welfare services, while the Global South has a predominance of the young, who lack employment opportunities and have little access to power. Among other consequences, this galvanizes migration flows of the young from the Global South to the Global North. This migrant inflow can be deployed to ease staff shortages – for instance, in agricultural labour and in health and social care sectors – or to take advantage of a 'brain drain' of the highly trained from the Global South, but it can and does also inflame opposition to migrants in parts of the Global North. In countries such as the UK, the national generational imbalance – a continuing decline in the size of the working population, following from lower birth rates, and an expansion of older age cohorts outside paid employment, caused by increased longevity – gives impetus not only to migration but to innovations that replace or supplement human labour by machines, to address labour shortages and sluggish productivity. So far so familiar. Replacing human labour by machine processes is very much what happened in each earlier Industrial Revolution. Some analysts, however, see the implications of AI as something new.

The AI revolution is already well underway. A small group of dominant tech entrepreneurs has called for a pause in the rollout of AI for fear of its potential dangers to humans, not the least of which is the ease with which AI can be used by almost anyone today with access to apps such as ChatGPT to spread fake news and invented 'facts'. Educationalists are currently putting pressure on media outlets such as YouTube to curb the spread of pseudoscience through what purport to be 'educational' programmes, and Hollywood script writers and actors have been on strike in the hope of constraining the use of AI to replace them and/or erode the level of their pay. Many science fiction and literary novels have been constructing their plots around imagining how AI and advanced technology may replace or radically alter humanity (see Ishiguro 2005, 2021). Yet most of the comments that fill the digital cloud, the mass media and the bookshops today are more concerned about who or, more accurately, which corporate entities will have control of AI and its applications for profit or power (Runciman 2023). In *The Age of Surveillance Capitalism*, Shoshana Zuboff's main target is the sinister side of AI and digital surveillance technology, particularly its potential to violate the privacy of the citizen consumer for the political benefit of governments and to swell the profits of big corporations (Zuboff 2019).

Who should control AI has been a central theme of recent BBC Reith Lectures. Stuart Russell's 2021 series warns about the potential dangers if humans fail to exert control over AI, the uses to which it is put and the likelihood of building systematic biases into its operation. In particular, Russell highlights the potential destructiveness of autonomous weapons systems (Russell 2021). The Reith Lectures of 2023 by Ben Ansell on 'Our democratic future' raise related themes. In the fourth lecture, on the future of prosperity, Ansell argues that it is important to have a democratic debate about how the tech companies can be effectively regulated; otherwise, they will have a virtual monopoly of the profits generated by the use of AI to raise productivity. This is far more urgent than imagining dystopian futures where machines control humans, especially if generative AI ever enables machines to 'think for themselves' (Ansell 2023).

In a detailed projection of these changes, Daniel Susskind argues that we need to prepare for 'a world without work' (Susskind 2020). His is one of the more extreme versions of the likely effects of technology, automation and AI on the world of employment. Stuart Russell agrees that it is likely to reduce the need for human labour and that if it is not managed wisely, AI could indeed impoverish human lives (Russell 2020; see also Suleyman and Bhaksar 2023). Yet Russell also notes that for 10,000 years most societies have 'used humans like robots' and that we could choose to use AI to meet unmet needs and enrich human lives. Technological change always has at least two faces.

While there is dispute about the magnitude of the change, there is wide agreement that these new technologies, especially AI, are likely to eliminate jobs as they replace human labour by technology, just as previous Industrial Revolutions did. It is already happening as computers can, for example, review vast arrays of facts far more quickly and comprehensively than was possible in the very recent past for individuals or even teams of humans in offices, libraries and archives. Computer programs today can, for instance, interrogate a DNA population database to identify the individuals susceptible to particular diseases or health threats, and do it as well or better, and certainly faster, than is possible using only the judgement of individual human analysts. Such AI-assisted processes will, in many cases, act as adjuncts to tasks performed by humans, as already happens in some hospital medicine, preventive epidemiology and development of drugs. The composition of the dataset to be used and the questions posed to it are still decisions made by human judgement, even if some computer scientists foresee a time when these decisions will also be taken by AI without human intervention. At the moment, however, humans still decide what algorithms and datasets suit their purpose and can discard them if they prove to be unsuited to the purpose: when the COVID-19 lockdowns made the typical school examination process impossible in 2021, algorithms drawn from the distribution of past GCSE and A level examination results in Britain were initially used to award grades to individual students, but this produced results that teachers and students regarded as so unfair that the Department for Education replaced them with teacher-assessed grades.

Daniel Susskind's central contention is that whereas in previous technological revolutions machines usually replaced manual tasks, the current technological revolution is more likely to impact skilled professional jobs, the middle-class occupations that constitute the knowledge economy and usually require higher education qualifications. In the First Industrial Revolution, complex tasks that drew on human judgement and 'know-how' were subdivided into their constituent parts so that human art and dexterity could be replaced by regular, repeatable, single tasks performed mechanically. Although certain artisan skills, such as hand spinning, were rendered obsolete (or eventually confined to the handmade luxury market), the number of new jobs generated by the change usually outnumbered those that were lost within a generation, although they normally went to a different group of workers. What Susskind regards as new in AI is the ability of technology to perform skilled cerebral work, to replace what Marx called 'workers by brain' – rather than 'workers by hand' – the educated middle classes, specifically those postwar educationally mobile professionals like myself, produced by the vastly expanded higher education system after the Second World War. Susskind predicts that the ultimate effect will be to transfer most economic 'productivity' gains, which may be very considerable, to the owners and controllers of the intelligent computers and other technology – the tech companies and their head officials, such as Elon Musk, Mark Zuckerberg, and a host of less visible corporate executives – and to swell the incomes of a tiny cadre of highly skilled workers creating programs, maintaining and improving the hardware and software and developing the underlying science of the system.

Susskind believes that the vast majority of jobs that will disappear in this process will leave society with two enormous problems: how to redistribute the wealth thus generated from the controllers of technology to the mass of the jobless population, the alternative being to risk potentially serious social unrest; and how to give the workless a purpose in life to replace what paid work has come to mean in modern times – income, status, self-worth, dignity, a recognized place in society and community, and meaningful activity. Susskind, in common with many others currently working on the idea, proposes a universal basic income, which he believes should be subject to everyone 'earning' the right to receive it through socially useful activities, notably volunteering. Susskind clearly thinks that this will provide the opportunity to correct some of the historic problems of inequality in the distribution of economic prosperity, including the failure to reward the unpaid caring that has always fallen disproportionately on women, to determine who gets to control the technologies that have generated this prosperity, and to tackle the problem of meaning, the issue of how to live well. All these 'opportunities' also pose serious practical and political problems about how to arrive at such recalibrations. Susskind is no more specific than Mike Savage about the route to this desirable goal.

Other commentators stop well short of predicting anything close to Daniel Susskind's 'world without work'. Mark Carney, for instance, suggests that no more than 10–15 per cent of middle-class jobs are at risk of being replaced by technological change in most advanced economies, though a range between 10 per cent and as much as 50 per cent has been suggested (Carney 2021, pp 458–9). In Carney's view, change will usually affect the nature of jobs rather than their complete replacement. He believes job losses will be comparable to the 10–20 per cent loss over long periods in the most exposed sectors during the three previous Industrial Revolutions. Like Susskind and others, however, he argues that such changes offer a challenge but also incentive and opportunity to correct the injustices exposed in recent crises.

Most observers, including Mark Carney and Daniel Susskind, agree that jobs that have been classified as needing cognitive skills are likely to be major losers to AI. Minouche Shafik, for instance, includes accountants and auditors, general operations managers, business services and administration managers, financial analysts and lawyers in her list of jobs likely to experience redundancies, alongside routine white-collar workers such as postal clerks, customer service and client information workers, cashiers, ticket clerks and bank tellers (Shafik 2021, p 105, Table 2). Many of the latter are the kind of routine white-collar activities that Stuart Russell describes as society using humans like robots, and many of them have already been moved offshore to places with lower labour costs. Offshore call centres are already using AI to alter voices speaking English with Asian or African accents to sound more Anglo-American. Academics, journalists, writers, actors and musicians may be offered stiff competition by the large language models of AI; universities already search out digital programs to identify plagiarism and, increasingly, to identify work composed not by students themselves but by AI. Professionals in these sectors alternately call for rules and controls to protect their work and are vigorously sceptical about AI's capacity for 'real' creativity. The first International AI Summit in November 2023 at Bletchley Park, initiated by UK Prime Minister Rishi Sunak and with US Vice-President Kamala Harris and Ursula von der Leyen, President of the European Commission, attending, issued a declaration, signed by 25 national leaders, resolving to address the risks of AI. The United Nations also declared its support for the establishment of an AI expert panel on the lines of the Intergovernmental Panel on Climate Change. The Summit also announced an intention to collaborate with national governments and tech companies in testing advanced AI models before and after they are rolled out by the leading tech companies, which are mostly based in the US.

Can new technologies solve the care crisis?

The position of care work in many of these expert projections is chronically ambiguous. For all Daniel Susskind's sympathy for the undervalued care sector and for the army of unpaid women carers, he half-implies that care might be covered, wholly or in part, by the volunteer work that could be required from the able-bodied under a new form of 'national service' in return for universal basic income. Others, however, see it as 'real' but currently under-rewarded work that will be in ever greater demand as the population ages. Such work will need to be rewarded by a price that recognizes its social and moral value in ways that economics, as traditionally practised, does not.

David Goodhart is one of the commentators who does not minimize the 'work' character or undervalue the skills of care work (Goodhart 2020). He deplores the way the rise of the 'cognitive elite' has 'demoted' the other two sectors – manual and technical hands-on work, and all the caring work – whose members now feel 'left behind', undervalued and under-rewarded. Goodhart believes that the care and health sectors are likely to prove the fastest-increasing part of the formal economy as the proportion of the population in the older age groups rise.

In a radio discussion in summer 2023 about the future of work, Goodhart argued that with the balance of employment sectors changing, adjustments need to be made to their relative rewards (Rajan 2023). White-collar and professional jobs, which currently constitute 35–40 per cent of formal employment, already include a substantial amount of 'uncreative' work that is currently 'over-rewarded' and may be done as well or better by technology. By comparison, health and social care contain a substantial proportion of 'Cinderella jobs' that most people regard as seriously under-rewarded in relation to the degree of effort and emotional intelligence they require. Healthcare ranges from extremely well-paid, high-status medical consultants to a majority of Cinderella jobs in the lower echelons. Goodhart projected that the health sector was likely to increase to 20–25 per cent of all formal employment over the next two to three decades. Goodhart and the other participants in the radio discussion argued vehemently that the levels and differentiations of economic rewards are not fixed and inevitable – that is, not 'scientifically' fixed by the 'laws' of economics – but rather a matter of choices – value preferences. Moreover, they argued that although there is often no career progression or status in the Cinderella jobs in health and social care, they can be emotionally satisfying and, as a sector, care jobs have done rather better than low-skilled male manual work, which has lost any sense of communal importance it may once have enjoyed. Even so, there is a reluctance on the part of male manual workers to move over into what are sometimes described as 'pink' jobs – women's work. 'Good work' is more than pay and chances of promotion; autonomy and dignity in work matter. The 'soft skills' required by care work are not obviously replaceable by AI, and large numbers of young people want work they find meaningful and that serves the greater good of society. The latter sentiment is well documented and puts another question mark over the claim by the authors of the Gen Z study (Katz et al 2021) that values have become dominantly self-centred.

The Japanese experience

It may be instructive to consider the Japanese experience in the care sector. The Japanese are currently trialling robotic adjuncts in care homes – for instance, providing robotic substitute pets to soothe the anxieties of the old or of dementia patients, robots to perform some of the more mechanical aspects of care, tech-assisted 'muscle suits' that help carers lift and move patients, robots to assist and encourage the old and disabled in exercise classes and ICT such as video technology for surveillance to detect falls or other hazards at times and in places where there are no human carers present (Voigt and König 2021; Sylvester 2023). So far, these technological aids are essentially adjuncts rather than replacements for human carers, but the Japanese are anxious to deploy technology to address acute staff shortages and high rates of burnout in care work, which are the result of an even more precipitous and prolonged decline in the birth rate leading to even worse generational imbalance than the Americans and Europeans face.

In Japan, those of working age, as well as the overall population, have been in decline for decades, and the Organisation for Economic Co-operation and Development predicts that the population of working age is likely to decline further, by 20 per cent between 2017 and 2040 (cited in World Economic Forum 2019). With almost a third of the population already aged 65 and over, Japan has been reluctant to abandon the ideal that families take care of the old, but is being forced to consider nontraditional alternatives. Young Japanese women in full-time employment increasingly reject marriage and motherhood rather than find themselves trapped by gender expectations considerably more constricting and burdensome for women than they are in Europe. The Japanese have always protected their culture from migration and are now pioneers in the use of AI in the health and care system partly in the hope of staving off resort to non-Japanese migrants to supply the shortfall in family carers. They also encourage older people, especially women over the age of 65, into care work. The use of technological devices, ICT more than robotics, seems to be effective in relieving some of the stress experienced by care workers by limiting the burden of record keeping, leaving more time for actual care. Yet the severe limitations of AI as a stand-alone substitute for human carers has led the Japanese government to do the unthinkable and encourage migration from Southeast Asian countries to work in the care workforce. Only a very few of the AI and ICT innovations in Japanese care are appearing in Britain so far, although a few care homes are interested in trying out robot pets. A 2021 report of The King's Fund found considerable resistance to such innovations among care workers and a dearth of initiatives from leadership in this sphere, though the authors of the report saw potential value in such developments if these obstacles could be surmounted (Maguire et al 2021).

Discussion

Arguments of the kind rehearsed earlier can be found every day on the blogosphere and in journalism as well as in economic and political analyses. Why do they apparently cut so little ice in practical politics and with employers in Britain? One of the consequences in sectors that already employ extensive technology has been to intensify the work of the people who still have jobs and even to lengthen working hours. The fear of redundancy, perhaps, makes many workers reluctant to protest against technologically driven increases in the length or intensity of work – delivery drivers and warehouse operatives working for online stores such as Amazon, or delivery drivers for companies like Deliveroo or those providing taxi services for companies such as Uber may well be cases of this kind. Only a minority of highly unionized groups, such as railway workers, can afford to strike against the imposition of labour replacement or labour-intensifying technology, and it is not clear for how long they will successfully do so as technology renders obsolete many of their artisan skills, not least driving trains, taxis or buses in an era of driverless vehicles.

It seems doubtful that most people in government or in the management of the economy have yet fully absorbed the size of the challenge current technological changes present. Despite frequent protestations from politicians that they 'get' the problem of carers being undervalued and under-rewarded, I see little or nothing to suggest that this has dislodged traditional economic and political assumptions as they affect decisions and actions. Political parties continue to appeal to economic growth as the only way to finance welfare spending and vie with each other in protesting their intention not to raise taxes. A revision of the tax system and its underlying rationale is long overdue, and without that governments are unlikely to be able to hold capital to account in any effective way that truly addresses the inequalities and moral discrepancies in the distribution of the national wealth (Collini 2023; Johnson 2023). A recalibration of the work we value and reward is nowhere in the plans of politicians. If it were, it is unlikely to be a vote winner. Indeed, five-year parliaments are not conducive to long-term programmes in any area of policy let alone for the crises in care and climate.

In the creation of the welfare state after the Second World War, there was a strong current among the public in favour of collective provision and pooling of risk and a good deal of cross-party collaboration. The incipient secularity of that time was not yet fully developed and public values were, perhaps, still more potently 'haunted' by Christianity than is now the case (Spencer 2016). The second great commandment was still lodged in the recesses of most people's memory and the Christian churches had not yet lost their moral authority when Archbishop William Temple was a weighty and influential figure in the background of the Beveridge reforms. Where should we look to find similarly powerful moral champions for the recalibration of value that we have seen advocated by technocrats of capitalism and academic analysts? It poses the same political problems that a real determination to halt man-made climate change poses. Even when a majority of the electorate is in principle convinced that the change is desirable, even essential, as soon as it requires immediate sacrifices of comfort, convenience or income, their votes can no longer be relied on, especially when the costs fall heavily on those sectors least able to bear them.

And where is the Christian church in all this? It would be comforting to think that there was still moral weight and practical influence in the example of Christians who do so much volunteering to help others by running their neighbours to the doctor's surgery or to hospital in the absence of buses; by running food banks for the sake of that substantial minority who struggle to feed themselves and their families – nurses and care workers among them; by providing warm spaces at a time when heating one's home is an impossible luxury for so many; by offering hospitality to refugees and those experiencing misfortune, addiction or homelessness; or by doing what they can to halt climate change. Secular folk do all this too. Indeed, there is quite a lot of that urge to offer care to others in the secular population, including among the young. And for all the hedonistic indulgence and the pleasure in the humiliation of others that fuels parts of the mass media, notably 'reality television' and digital social media, there is also a continuing appetite for doing good, as witnessed by the willingness of the public to give to GoFundMe appeals on behalf of unfortunate individuals or families, or to contribute to large-scale fundraising appeals such as the BBC's yearly Children in Need, or to the BBC's DIY SOS Big Build projects, where local volunteers supply the materials and labour to build houses, youth centres and the like. Doing good for others still gets a pretty good press in Britain's secular popular culture, particularly when the others being helped are near to home and like us. Appeals by international charities for distant and 'foreign' others fare less well.

Unhappily, the churches are at least as much in the public consciousness for their internecine wars over sexuality as they are respected for reaching out to the vulnerable. Church leaders in Britain gallantly continue to challenge government penny-pinching and perverse economic priorities that weaken the care system and other parts of the welfare state because fairness cannot be 'afforded'. But their political impact is small. A young professional footballer or a pop or media star carries more cultural clout today than a bishop. With the collapse of Christian socialization, very few minds are still furnished with memories of the second great commandment, and Christian hauntings need *something* to prompt them. A society so fundamentally shaped by instrumental values, status competition and a toxic brew of hedonism and exaggerated individualism is not best placed to find the values that can motivate and support the political and economic changes that might begin to tackle the care crisis or the climate emergency. It is mildly astonishing that so many in the British population show altruistic impulses as strongly as they do.

After the Second World War, structural crises made it possible for postwar governments across Europe to create welfare states. The redistributive tax policies that made that a reality had the mass support of populations wearied by war and privation, longing for a better deal in the peace, something that had not happened despite the political promises after the Great War. There was a groundswell of public opinion on which these policies could be successfully floated, despite postwar austerity as Europe began to pay its vast war debt to the mighty US. There was an active Christian component in that groundswell as well as among the political class. This meant that support for the NHS and the rest of the postwar welfare settlement could not plausibly be represented as popular communism or emulation of the USSR, which, with 'Uncle Joe' Stalin, began to alter in the popular mind from wartime ally to totalitarian threat soon after the war ended. Winston Churchill tried but failed to make support for the Labour Party look like support for totalitarian socialism in the 1945 election campaign. Christian principles of care for one's neighbour were important enough elements in the mix to ensure that the Labour Party and the British welfare settlement were never seen as alien ideological innovations by the great majority of the electorate.

Today, the Christian input is still there but it resonates less strongly in the general population and has insufficient weight to inspire the radical, perhaps even sacrificial, policies that will be necessary to throw 'growth at all costs' from its policy throne and deliver the care sector and the climate from looming disaster which is already hitting the poorest and most marginalized hardest and first. Perhaps the radical changes heralded by AI and the rest of the Fourth Industrial Revolution will indeed render radical change necessary, although a crisis of mass worklessness is hardly something to be wished for as a spur. Yet the policies that such radical change will require cannot happen without power, moral conviction and a commitment to the public good. And, at least in immediate terms, it will call for *political* courage, as it will mean finding ways of redistributing some of the excessive spoils of capitalism from a small elite to the wider community rather than following politics and economics 'as usual' and the siren appeal of realpolitik and personal ambition.

But the impossible and unlikely *do* occur; and hope is not only a Christian virtue but a human necessity.

I am unlikely to live long enough to see what happens to the problems that have engaged me in this book, but I hope we may find somewhere within us all, politicians and citizens alike, the kindness for the distant stranger as well as the immediate neighbour, for the folk we don't know personally who live in potentially uninhabitable parts of the world menaced by climate change, for the disreputable prodigals in our own communities and for the poor, sick, disabled and simply old who need help to live well.

Notes

Chapter 1

1 A normal school trained teachers for elementary school teaching and many of them subsequently became regular teacher training colleges. Teaching younger children was usually part of the training.

2 She organized and directed a burglary of her parents' home to fund the IRA and later spent time in prison for her active role in the bombing of a barracks.

3 Many of the terraces in the town where my family lived were eventually improved and modernized rather than demolished and replaced by high-rise flats as happened in the central areas of Manchester and Salford photographed by Shirley Baker. The streets of my childhood are now largely occupied by ethnic minority communities and the redundant Nonconformist chapels now serve as mosques and Muslim community halls. Selections of Baker's street photographs, which vividly catch the spirit of communities from the 1960s to the 1980s, were widely exhibited throughout the North West during her lifetime and shown shortly after her death in her first solo exhibition, 'Women and children; and loitering men', in 2015, first in The Photographers' Gallery in London and then in a worldwide tour.

4 When I read Parsons' theoretical works for myself, I found that while it is possible to extrapolate such an argument from his functional theories of the social system, his early essays on the social psychology of the family and on the emergence of the nuclear family in modernity are more concerned to argue that working-class fathers have little power to advance their sons into middle-class occupations than to make an explicit argument about the rivalry between fathers and sons as an explanation for the dominance of the nuclear family in mobile modern social systems.

Chapter 2

1 Howard Jacobson refers to this common anti-semitic usage in the eloquent, funny, sad memoir of his boyhood in the Jewish community of Cheetham Hill, Manchester, a few miles down the road from the gentile community in which I grew up (Jacobson 2022). He describes his embarrassment at having to spend his weekends and school holidays on his father's market stall all over the North West, mortified at being the sidekick in the sales patter and jokes. According to Julia Boyd, the usage, sometimes expressed as 'to jew down', in the sense of driving down a price or making an advantageous bargain, was unselfconsciously used by all classes and was still current, although culturally tabooed, among some Americans as recently as 2013 (Boyd 2017, p 132).

2 Some of these Whit processions incorporated a 'Christianized' folk celebration of the May Queen in the guise of Mary.

3 The literature is extensive but some accounts summarize the general picture (Bruce 1995, 2011, 2021; Woodhead and Catto 2012; Davie 2015), though they differ in their interpretation of the data. A sequence of books by Clive Field over the last few years sets

out the definitive statistical picture of British secularization, based on material accumulated over a lifetime's research and previously published piecemeal (Field 2015, 2017, 2019, 2021). See also the review essay on all four of Field's volumes (Bruce 2022; see also Bruce and Voas 2023).

4 There is a whole literature on theories of the modern (integrated) and the postmodern (fragmented) self, which need not detain us here. But for a superbly economical discussion of this whole problem, see Terry Eagleton's critique of the implications of current narrative conceptions of the self: (Eagleton 2023).

5 Shamima Begum was married to an ISIS fighter at age 16 in the caliphate and gave birth to three children, all of whom died as babies under the privations of civil war.

6 An exhibition of pictures and other artworks representing St Francis was held in the reopened National Portrait Gallery in July 2023. It included part of an altarpiece by Sassetta – originally made for the San Sepolcro friary but now in the permanent collection of The National Gallery, London – which depicts the naked Francis renouncing his privilege by piling his rich clothing at his disapproving father's feet. Giotto has a similar treatment of the occasion in his frescoes in Assisi. There are many stories and some pictures of Francis stripping off his clothes to give to a poor knight and to a beggar.

7 There is a good deal of criticism of the way religious education is taught in schools. Critical Ofsted reports in 2013, 2017 and 2021 suggest it is often superficial or misleading and fails to prepare students for a multi-religious and secular society (Davies 2021, p 4).

8 This issue also affects the methodology of the physical sciences where in quantum mechanics the observer alters the behaviour of particles at the atomic and subatomic level. Wendy Brown discusses some of these problems in *Nihilistic Times*, in which she analyses the intellectual tradition of strict demarcation between disciplines in academic life and between political and intellectual perspectives, focusing on Max Weber's distinction between fact and value (Brown 2023). The erosion of these strict boundaries in later 20th-century culture is what she designates as 'nihilism'. See also the review of her book by William Davies (Davies 2023, p 11). These issues occur in current 'identity politics' (discussed in the following chapter) as well as in the secularization of the universities and the way they have become political arenas. The classical insistence on 'methodological agnosticism' in the sociology of religion and even in some academic theology, which requires the scholar to suspend any religious, moral or political conviction and remain untouched by affect, has been weakened in the course of the 21st century. For a thoughtful and incisive treatment of the issue in the sociology of religion, see Mathew Guest's *Neoliberal Religion*, particularly its impressive final chapter (Guest 2022).

Chapter 3

1 I am indebted to Grace Davie for this information.

2 It is, of course, impossible to know just how influential the years of Sunday school actually were in the construction of Larry Henry's sensibility. The same would be true of the boyhood of the broadcaster Clive Myrie, who has made television programmes about his family's Catholic community in Jamaica and later in Bolton.

3 I am grateful to Grace Davie for this reference.

4 David Goodhart distinguishes between 'Anywheres' and 'Somewheres', which roughly parallels the liberal/ethnocentric distinction of Kolpinskaya and Fox, but without taking account of religious variables (Goodhart 2017).

5 I am indebted to Mathew Guest for pointing out this contrast and its political and social implications.

Chapter 4

1 Daniels' article is generally agreed to be the first usage of the term which was subsequently widely adopted in feminist arguments.

2 Adapted with modern twists by Richard Bean and Oliver Chris, *Jack Absolute Flies Again*, loosely based on Sheridan's *The Rivals*, was performed in summer 2022 at the National Theatre, London. The setting in 2022 is an airfield during the Battle of Britain, and Lydia Languish has become a feminist woman pilot delivering replacement Spitfires to the airfield instead of a dreamy young woman living in her imagination in a romantic novel. The anachronism is, presumably, a deliberate joke. The sexual jokes are post sexual revolution and the whole play has shifted very far from the evangelical narrative and even from the sexual norms of the 1940s, even though war was loosening many older taboos. The impact of the new play depends on a knowing audience reading the ironies by comparing the new version with Sheridan's original and its expected 'happy ending', which is aborted in the new version by Jack Absolute's heroic death in the Battle of Britain.

3 Barbara Pym, a novelist of the 1950s and 1960s, is described by her most recent biographer as incessantly looking for love but not marriage. As a young woman, Pym loved Richardson's *Pamela*, but abruptly lost interest 'when Mr B's intentions towards his beautiful maidservant became honourable' (Byrne 2021, p 3). Pym wrote half-melancholy, witty comedies about women like herself – frustrated, respectable, usually churchgoing, genteelly fading and still half-longing for love affairs – while casting a sardonic eye on the failings of men and the unsatisfactory marriages she observes. Her novels went out of favour in the later 1960s as sexual mores altered and what was made explicit in novels expanded. Pym's work and its reception (more accurately, the judgement of her publisher about its marketability) mark the transition in the gender order. Pym's final, darker-toned novels were only published at the end of the 1970s after she was 'rediscovered' by Lord David Cecil in *The Times Literary Supplement*, after nearly two decades of unsuccessful advocacy by Philip Larkin.

4 Deborah Orr describes abortion rather than contraception as the usual resort of university students in the 1980s and gives an account of the sexual culture she experienced as strikingly similar to what is only today being publicly castigated as a popular 'rape culture', fed by the pornography so easily available to today's internet generations (Orr 2020); Jessica Martin paints a similar picture of the often exploitative sexual culture and gendered moral standards of the 1980s (Martin 2020); Paula Byrne's biography of Barbara Pym implies that much the same was already true of Oxford student life for women in the early 1930s (Byrne 2020); and the documentary on the life and work of the artist Paula Rego by Nick Willing, her son, shows abortion as routine among the young women students at the Slade School of Art in the mid-1930s (Willing 2017). See also Elizabeth Roberts' *Women and Families* (Roberts 1995); Lorna Finlayson's review of *Complaint!* by Sarah Ahmed, about the MeToo movement, which discusses the prevalence of sexual violence and harassment against women and the inadequacies of complaints procedures in Britain's 'marketized' universities (Finlayson 2022). See also: Jean McCrindle and Sheila Rowbotham's *Dutiful Daughters*, which documents the widespread ignorance among both women and men about sexuality, which the Women's Liberation Movement hoped to rectify (McCrindle and Rowbotham 1977); a history of unmarried mothers in Britain (Thane and Evans 2012); and an Ofsted report published in June 2021 documenting a high incidence of sexual harassment, including rape, reported by female school pupils at the hands of male fellow students, fed by the easy availability of often violent pornography from a very young age (Ofsted 2021).

5 Examples are scattered through Margaretta Jolly's history of the Women's Liberation Movement in Britain (Jolly 2019). The argument was often aired through popular

culture – for instance, in Malcolm Bradbury's redbrick campus novel *The History Man*, which focuses on a charismatic don, Howard Kirk, in a satire on the misogynist 1970s radical (Bradbury 1975). The novel was adapted for the BBC in 1981 and became a popular series.

6 In Europe, marriage had traditionally been a family and civic matter and only began to be regarded as a sacrament by the church in the 12th century, a position that was made official only in 1563 by the Council of Trent as part of the contest with the Reformers. The parallel interest of state and church in the institution of marriage has played out ever since that time.

7 Brockes' Passion libretto (1712) was a dramatic, quasi-romantic poetic version of Christ's Passion in the German language, which was set as an oratorio by a number of composers including Telemann, and, most famously, Handel in 1719, early in his career in Munich. Poems by Brockes that vividly illustrate the transition of devotional poetry towards Romanticism in their paeons to the Creator of Nature were used in *Neun deusche Arien*, composed by Handel between 1724 and 1726.

Chapter 5

1 She discusses the significance of these fantasy books for children in a book on the Eucharist (Martin 2023, pp 77–85).

2 This is not only linked to the colloquial use of 'dirty Arab' in working-class Lancashire to describe boys whose skin is discoloured with dirt or their clothes are dishevelled, but it also supports Kenan Malik's analysis of the significance of racist perceptions in his discussion of when and why the British working class came to be described as 'White' (see Chapter 2).

3 A celebrated painting from about 1850, *Found Drowned*, by G. F. Watts in the Watts Gallery, Compton, Surrey, shows a young pregnant woman who has jumped from Waterloo Bridge into the Thames. It was painted in response to the poem 'Bridge of Sighs' by Thomas Hood, illustrating an everyday London tragedy.

4 One of the Chilean Methodist Pentecostal pastors whom my husband and I interviewed in Chile in the early 1990s did the same thing, learning his letters by memorizing the first letter of each of the surnames of the labourers as he looked at the overseer's list as the men were given their pay on the estate where he worked as a boy.

5 The eldest son of Grace Davie was given *Her Benny* as a reading book in his primary school in Liverpool as late as the 1980s.

6 Orsi presented some of his evidence to a seminar at the London School of Economics and Political Science in autumn 2020.

Chapter 6

1 Alison Light points out that modern editors of *Aurora Leigh* (Barrett-Browning nd; discussed in Chapter 4) have seen it as a 'secular vision of New Jerusalem formed in the new dawn of more equal relations between women and men' (Light 2022, p 87).

2 Alison Light offers a succinct critique of the tendency of some male poets and critics to infantilize Rossetti as 'childlike' and 'sentimental' without seeing the ambiguities in her version of Victorian womanliness in her poetry (Light 2022, pp 83, 85, 89).

3 Much of this oeuvre is on display in Tate Britain, London, including Spencer's painting of his father as St Francis of Assisi feeding the birds in the Spencer family farmyard.

4 It is unclear how far, as an adult, Maeve Gilmore remained a practising Roman Catholic, but she had been educated in a convent school, married in a Roman Catholic Church and had her children baptized, as she records in her memoir of her life with Mervyn Peake. He had a Dissenting upbringing as the son of a medical missionary in China.

Their life together was classically bohemian. In the moving conclusion of her memoir, Gilmore grieves for her husband's decline in his mid-forties into what his doctor called 'premature senility' as a result of Parkinson's disease. As she visits his physical shell in the care home, she laments the loss not only of her husband but of God. She writes: 'I've forgotten about God. Once he was part of our universe, but he has gone, and the thin line has gone, and there is nothing left but what I know of you. Dark man ... Funny man ... Gentle man. Man that made something new each day. Where are you? Please tell me where you have gone' (Gilmore 1970, p 140).

5 A video of the murals, recorded before the new owners of the house had them painted out, can be accessed on the Instagram archive of Gilmore's work (Peake nd).

6 Tomalin gives an account of Dickens' mid-life repudiation of his wife, Catherine, and his close relationship first with her sister Mary, who lived with them and died young, and then with her sister Georgina, who effectively became Dickens' lifelong housekeeper and confidante, as well as his secret affair with the actress Ellen Ternan (Tomalin 2012). These episodes have provided good copy for contemporary writers, who can now openly discuss attitudes and behaviour hidden under a cloak of respectability and to which the Victorians would often have turned a blind eye, especially in 'a great man'. The celebrated Australian novelist Peter Carey uses a fictionalized Dickens, Tobias Oates, in his novel *Jack Maggs* – Carey's reimagined version of the convict, Magwich, from *Great Expectations* – to embody Dickens' ruthless manipulation of others, his self-dramatization, his colonial prejudices and his sexual double standards (Carey 1997).

7 Early trade union struggles often had to face the absence of legal protection for collective rather than individual 'persons' in English common law – for example, if their funds were embezzled or stolen or their collective rights were breached or denied. The struggle for legal protection of 'corporate persons' continued for over a century.

8 See also an imaginative novel on the view 'from downstairs', including the feelings of the servants about the drudgery that it fell to them to perform for their 'betters', the bestselling novel *Longbourn* by Jo Baker (Baker 2013). It gives an account of the lives of the servants of the Bennett family in Jane Austen's classic story *Pride and Prejudice*.

9 Virginia Woolf's, 'introductory letter' in *Life as We Have Known It: The Voices of Working Class Women*, edited by Margaret Llewelyn Davies, was reprinted by Virago in 2012. In 1913 Virginia Woolf had attended a meeting of the Co-operative Women's Society with her husband, Leonard, who was a supporter of the Co-operative Movement, and even though she formally joined the society, and gave a series of lectures for working people at Morley College in the early 1930s, much of the introductory letter is based on that single experience.

10 Hermione Lee gives considerable attention to the possibility that her distaste for the body could stem from Virginia Stephen probably having been sexually molested by one or more of her older Duckworth stepbrothers from her mother's first marriage (Lee 2007).

11 Under the Factory and Workshops Act 1901, 'half-timers' were pupils who had reached the educational standard expected for school leavers by age 12 and were allowed to work for half the day for the rest of their time in compulsory education. They alternated school and work, one week school in the morning and the mill in the afternoon, then vice versa the following week. My aunts used to tell me how they would regularly fall asleep on their desks on afternoons when they had been 'on mornings in the mill'.

12 Harriet Vane is used by Sayers to mount a critique of the culture of respectability and the prevalent double standard of sexual morality. Harriet is given a back history, beginning in the novel *Strong Poison*, where she is tried for the murder of her bohemian lover. Vane is only saved by the investigations of Peter Wimsey, who proves her innocence and begins an importunate pursuit to get her to marry him. This takes the two of them through

several subsequent crime novels of which *Gaudy Night* is the penultimate one. Harriet Vane, unlike Dorothy Sayers, her creator, is given no living parents to be scandalized by her sexual history.

13 I thank my daughter, Jessica Martin, for reminding me of the aptness of this Dorothy Sayers novel and I am indebted to her for her contribution to the argument in this chapter through her essay and in several conversations (Martin 2019).

14 The term 'intersectionality' was first used by an American legal scholar Kimberlé Crenshaw in the late 1980s in analysing the complexities of social justice, but it was later taken up more widely in the social sciences, especially in the 21st century, to do justice to the interrelations of what had often been discussed as self-contained systems of 'oppression', such as gender, race or class, which often reinforce each other as intensified layers of marginality.

15 This often occurs in studies of Pentecostalism in the Global South that document the sectional power or agency of women in the movement despite their general racial, class and gender inequality and their exclusion from formal leadership in church. See, for example, Judith Casselberry and Elizabeth A. Pritchard's *Spirit on the Move* and Christy K. Schuetze's *Spirit Wives and Church Mothers* (Casselberry and Pritchard 2019; Schuezte 2023). Schuezte emphasizes the way women in her study do not actively seek independent 'empowerment' but prioritize the welfare and stability of the family.

16 Muriel Spark's short story 'You should have seen the mess!' plays on the outrage of a nice working-class girl who works for middle-class families not unlike the Samuels. In an analysis of the counterculture published at the beginning of the 1980s, I used Spark's story to contrast the ideal of domestic orderliness among the 'respectable' working class with, on the one hand, the 'feckless' poor from whom they needed urgently to differentiate themselves and, on the other hand, the middle-class bohemians I only began to meet for the first time when I joined the middle classes myself as a university teacher (Martin 1981, pp 54–5).

17 One of the letters I received in response to this piece was from a young man from the Manchester area asking, rhetorically, how I knew his family so well and wondering whether I understood why he needed to escape from the domestic tyranny of northern women. I later developed this framework in work on the ambiguities in unequal gender roles in Pentecostalism in the Global South (Martin 2001, 2013).

18 I am indebted to Grace Davie for drawing the latter observation to my attention.

Chapter 8

1 The Post Office scandal of 2023 on is likely to be cited in management textbooks yet to be written as an example of many of the dysfunctions that Davies analyses, notably decrebration and the violation of Ashby's principle (or perhaps as something worse).

References

Abercrombie, Nicholas, Baker, John, Brett, Sebastian, and Foster, Jane (1970) 'Superstition and religion: the God of the gaps', in Martin, D. and Hill, M. (eds) *A Sociological Yearbook of English Religion*, London: SCM, pp 93–129.

Abrams, Lynn (2013) 'Mothers and daughters: negotiating the discourse on the "good woman" in 1950s and 1960s Britain', in Christie, Nancy, and Gavreau, Michael (eds) *The Sixties and Beyond: Dechristianisation in Western Europe and North America*, Toronto: University of Toronto Press, pp 60–83.

Ahmed, Athar (2021) *Life Chances*, BBC Radio 4. www.bbc.co.uk/programmes/m000s7mq

Alvaredo, Facundo, Chancel, Lucas, Piketty, Thomas, Saez, Emmanuel, and Lucman, Gabriel (eds) (2018) *World Inequality Report 2018*, Cambridge MA: Harvard University Press.

Alzheimer's Research UK (nd) 'Dementia statistics hub'. www.dementiastatistics.org

Ammerman, Nancy, and Davie, Grace (2019) '"A lived, situated and constantly changing reality": why religion is relevant to the pursuit of social progress', *International Panel on Social Progress*, Chapter 16.

Ansell, Ben (2023) 'The future of prosperity', The Reith Lectures on 'Our Democratic Future', Lecture 4, BBC Radio 4. www.bbc.co.uk/programmes/m001thz1

Archbishops' Commission on Reimagining Care (2023) *Care and Support Reimagined*. www.churchofengland.org/about/archbishops-commissions/reimagining-care-commission

Baker, Jo (2013) *Longbourne*, London: Doubleday.

Baker, Shirley (2018) *Without a Trace: Manchester and Salford in the 1960s*, Cheltenham: The History Press.

Barker, Kate (2014) *A New Settlement for Health and Social Care*, The King's Fund. www.kingsfund.org.uk/insight-and-analysis/reports/new-settlement-health-social-care-final-report#:~:text=The%20commission%2C%20chaired%20by%20Kate,towards%20the%20end%20of%20life

Barnett, Emma, and Peake, Christian (2022) Interview with Christian Peake on Woman's Hour, BBC Radio 4, 15 June. www.bbc.co.uk/sounds/play/m00187wx

Barrett Browning, Elizabeth (nd) 'Aurora Leigh', in *The Poetical Works of Elizabeth Barrett Browning*, Edinburgh: W.T. Nimmo, Hay and Mitchell, pp 562–749.

Barry, Sebastian (2023) *Old God's Time*, London: Faber.

BBC News (2023) 'Teesside care sector abuse and neglect concerns rise', 3 February. www.bbc.co.uk/news/uk-england-tees-55915891

Bennett, A.E. (1901/2018) *Fame and Fiction: An Enquiry into Certain Popularities* (Digital reprint), London: Forgotten Books.

Blackburn, Robert M., and Jarman, Jennifer (1993) 'Changing inequalities in access to British universities', *Oxford Review of Education*, 19(2): 197–215.

Blair, Tony (2023) (Quoted Brian Wheeler). www.bbc.co.uk/news/uk-politics-27112774

Bolton, Paul (2024) 'Higher education student numbers', House of Commons Library. https://researchbriefings.files.parliament.uk/documents/CBP-7857/CBP-7857.pdf

Boyd, Julia (2017) *Travellers in the Third Reich: The Rise of Fascism through the Eyes of Everyday People*, London: Elliott and Thompson.

Bradbury, Malcolm (1975) *The History Man*, London: Picador.

Bradstock, Andrew (2019) *David Sheppard: Batting for the Poor*, London: SCM.

Bregman, Rutger (2020) *Humankind: A Hopeful History*, London: Bloomsbury.

Brewitt-Taylor, Sam (2013) 'The invention of a "secular society"? Christianity and the sudden appearance of secularisation discourses in the British media, 1960–64', *Twentieth-Century British History*, 24(3): 327–50.

Brewitt-Taylor, Sam (2018) *Christian Radicalism in the Church of England and the Invention of the British Sixties 1957–1970: The Hope of a World Transformed*, Oxford: Oxford University Press.

British Medical Association (2024) 'NHS backlog data analysis'. www.bma.org.uk/advice-and-support/nhs-delivery-and-workforce/pressures/nhs-backlog-data-analysis

Brown, Andrew, and Woodhead, Linda (2016) *That Was the Church that Was: How the Church of England Lost the English People*, London: Bloomsbury.

Brown, Callum G. (2001) *The Death of Christian Britain: Understanding Secularisation 1800–2000*, Abingdon: Routledge.

Brown, Callum G. (2013) 'Gender, Christianity and the rise of no-religion: the heritage of the sixties in Britain', in Christie, Nancy, and Gavreau, Michael (eds) *The Sixties and Beyond: Dechristianization in North America and Western Europe*, Toronto: University of Toronto Press, pp 39–59.

Brown, Callum G. (2016) 'Unfettering religion: women and the family chain', *Studies in Church History*, 50: 469–91.

Brown, Callum G. (2017) *Becoming Atheist: Humanism and the Secular West*, London: Bloomsbury.

Brown, Callum G. (2019) *The Battle for Christian Britain: Sex, Humanists and Secularisation 1945–1980*, Cambridge: Cambridge University Press.

Brown, Roger, and Carasso, Helen (2913) *Everything for Sale? The Marketisation of Higher Education*, London: Routledge.

Brown, Wendy (2023) *Nihilistic Times: Thinking with Max Weber*, Cambridge MA: Harvard University Press.

Browne, Sarah (2013) 'Women, religion and the turn to feminism: experiences of Women's liberation activists in Britain in the seventies', in Christie, Nancy, and Gavreau, Michael (eds) in *The Sixties and Beyond: Dechristicnization in Western Europe and North America*, Toronto: University of Toronto Press, pp 84–97.

Bruce, Steve (1995) *Religion in Modern Britain*, Oxford: Oxford University Press.

Bruce, Steve (2011) *Secularization: In Defence of an Unfashionable Theory*, Oxford: Oxford University Press.

Bruce, Steve (2014) *Scottish Gods*, Edinburgh: Edinburgh University Press.

Bruce, Steve (2020) *British Gods: Religion in Modern Britain*, Oxford: Oxford University Press.

Bruce, Steve (2022) 'Mapping religious change in the UK: the work of Clive Field', *Journal of Contemporary Religion*, 17(2): 357–61.

Bruce, Steve, and Voas, David (2023) 'Secularization vindicated', *Religions*, 14(3): art 301. www.mdpi.com/2077-1444/14/3/301t

Bukodi, Erzsébet, and Goldthorpe, John (2018) *Social Mobility and Education in Britain*, Cambridge: Cambridge University Press.

Bunting, Madeleine (2020) *Labours of Love: The Crisis of Care*, London: Granta.

Burns, Jim (2013) *The History and Memories of the Whit Walks: In and around the Manchester Area with Banners and Bands*, Birkenhead: Countywise Ltd.

Butler, James (2023) 'This concerns everyone', *London Review of Books*, 45(5): 11–15.

Byrne, Paula (2021) *The Adventures of Miss Barbara Pym*, London: Harper Collins.

Carey, John (1992) *The Intellectuals and the Masses: Pride and Prejudice among the Literary Intellectuals, 1880–1939*, London: Faber.

Carey, Peter (1997) *Jack Maggs*, London: Faber.

Carney, Mark (2021) *Value(s): Building a Better World for All*, London: William Collins.

Carney, Mark (2023) The Reith Lectures on 'How We Get What We Value', BBC Radio 4. www.bbc.co.uk/programmes/m000py8v

Casselberry, Judith, and Pritchard, Elizabeth A. (eds) (2019) *Spirit on the Move: Pentecostalism and Black Women in Africa and the Diaspora*, Durham, NC: Duke University Press.

Cavendish, Camilla (2013) *The Cavendish Review: An Independent Review into the Healthcare Assistants and Support Workers in the NHS and Social Care Settings*. https://assets.publishing.service.gov.uk/media/5a7b9df6e5274a7202e18537/Cavendish_Review.pdf

Census 2021 (2021) 'Births, deaths and marriages', Office for National Statistics. https://www.ons.gov.uk/peoplepopulationandcommunity/birthsdeathsandmarriages

Christie, Nancy, and Gavreau, Michael (2013) 'Introduction', in Christie, Nancy, and Gavreau, Michael (eds) *The Sixties and Beyond: Dechristianization in Western Europe and North America*, Toronto: University of Toronto Press, pp 60–83.

Christophers, Brett (2023) *Our Lives in their Portfolios: Why Asset Managers Own the World*, London: Verso.

Clements, Ben (2017) 'How religious groups voted in the 2016 referendum on Britain's EU membership', *British Religion in Numbers*, 11 May. www.brin.ac.uk/how-religious-groups-voted-at-the-2016-referendum-on-britains-eu-membership/

Clery, E.J. (2004) *The Feminization Debate in Eighteenth-Century English Literature: Literature, Commerce and Luxury*, Basingstoke: Palgrave Macmillan.

Coles, Richard (2015) *Fathomless Riches: Or How I Went from Pop to Pulpit*, London: Weidenfeld and Nicolson.

Coles, Richard (2021) *The Madness of Grief: A Memoir of Love and Loss*, London: Weidenfeld and Nicolson.

Collini, Stefan (2012) *What Are Universities For?* London: Penguin.

Collini, Stefan (2018) 'The marketisation of higher education', *Fabian Society*, 22 February. https://fabians.org.uk/the-marketisation-of-higher-education/

Collini, Stefan (2023) 'Where to draw the line', *London Review of Books*, 45(20): 15–18.

Commission on Funding of Care and Support (2011) *Fairer Care Funding: The Report of the Commission on Funding of Care and Support*. https://webarchive.nationalarchives.gov.uk/ukgwa/20130221121534/http://www.dilnotcommission.dh.gov.uk/our-report/

Connolly, Billy (2020) *Billy Connolly: Portrait of a Lifetime*, Documentary, BBC Four, 9 August.

Cooper, Thia (2021) *Queer and Indecent: An Introduction to Marcella Althaus-Reid*, London, SCM.

Cottrell-Boyce, Frank (2012) 'London 2012: opening ceremony saw all our mad dreams come true', *The Guardian*, 29 July. www.theguardian.com/commentisfree/2012/jul/29/frank-cottrell-boyce-olympics-opening-ceremony

D'Ancona, Matthew (2021) *Identity, Ignorance, Innovation: Why the Old Politics Is Useless*, London: Hodder and Stoughton.

Daniels, Arlene Kaplan (1987) 'Invisible work', *Social Problems*, 14(3): 403–14.

Davenport, Bob (2015) 'Silas K. Hocking: author and minister', *Studies Monuments*. www.studiedmonuments.wordpress.com/2015/08/07silas-k-hocking-author-and-minister

Davie, Grace (2006) 'Vicarious religion: a methodological challenge', in Ammerman, Nancy (ed) *Everyday Religion: Observing Modern Religious Lives*, Oxford: Oxford University Press, pp 21–35.

Davie, Grace (2015) *Religion in Britain: A Persistent Paradox* (2nd edn), Oxford: Wiley-Blackwell.

Davie, Grace (2017) *Religion in Public Life: Levelling the Ground*, London: Theos and Edmund Cadbury Centre for the Understanding of Religion.

Davie, Grace (2022) 'Religion, secularity and secularization in Europe', in Davie, Grace, and Leustean, Lucian N. (eds) *The Oxford Handbook of Religion in Europe*, Oxford: Oxford University Press, pp 268–86.

Davie, Grace, and Ammerman, Nancy (2019) 'Why religion is relevant to the pursuit of social progress', in *ICSP (International Panel on Social Progress) Report*, Chapter 16.

Davies, Dan (2024) *The Unaccountability Machine: Why Big Systems Make Terrible Decisions – and How the World Lost its Mind*, London: Polity.

Davies, Madeleine (2021) 'RE teaching falls short of Ofsted's standards', *The Church Times*, 14 May, p 4.

Davies, William (2022) 'Stay away from politics' (Review of Wendy Brown, *Nihilistic Times*), *London Review of Books*, 45(18).

Davies, William (2023) 'Pain, no gain! William Davies on changing political economy', *London Review of Books*, 45(17): 7–10.

Day, Abby, and Lee, Lois (2014) 'Making sense of surveys and censuses: issues in religious self-identification', *Religion*, 40(14): 345–56.

de Araujo, Juan (2005) 'Aqui, aqui, valentones!' (audio CD) in Ex Cathedra and Geoffrey Skidmore (artists), *Baroque Music from Latin America (volume 2): Moon, Sun and All Things*, Hyperion.

De Bellaigue, Christina, Worth, Eva, Bennett, Charlotte, Eli, Karen, and Ulijaszek, Stanley (2022) 'Women, mobility and education in twentieth-century England and Wales: a new analytic approach', *Twentieth-Century History*, 33(3): 345–68.

Delap, Lucy (2011) *Knowing their Place: Domestic Servants in Twentieth-Century Britain*, Oxford: Oxford University Press.

Delap, Lucy (2020) *Feminisms: A Global History*, London: Pelican.

Department for Education (2022) 'Academic year 2021/22: Schools, pupils and their characteristics', *GOV.UK*. https://explore-education-statistics.service.gov.uk/find-statistics/school-pupils-and-their-characteristics

Department for Education (2024) 'Academic year 2023/24: schools, pupils and their characteristics', *GOV.UK*. https://explore-education-statistics.service.gov.uk/find-statistics/school-pupils-and-their-characteristics

Desmond, Matthew (2023) *Poverty, by America*, London: Allen Lane.

Donovan, Patrick (2022) *Arnold Bennett: Lost Idol*, Lewes: Unicorn.

Douglas, Ann (1977) *The Feminization of American Culture*, New York: Knopf.

Dowling, Emma (2022) *The Care Crisis: What Caused It and How We Can End It*, London: Verso.

Drabble, Margaret (1986) *Arnold Bennett: A Biography*, Boston, MA: G.K. Hall and Co.

Drabble, Margaret (2022) 'A writer with class', *Times Literary Supplement*, 6215: 3–4.

Eagleton, Terry (2022) 'What's Your Story?' (Review of Peter Brooks, *Seduced by Story: The Use and Abuse of Narrative*), *London Review of Books*, 45(4): 29–30.

Explore Education Statistics (characteristics of school students – ethnicity) (2023–4). https://explore-education-statistics.service.gov.uk/find-statistics/school-pupils-and-their-characteristics

El-Erian, Mohamad and Mazzucato, Mariana (2023) Interview with Victoria Derbyshire, *Newsnight*, BBC Two, 23 November.

Field, Clive (2015) *Britain's Last Religious Revival? Quantifying Believing, Behaving and Belonging in the Long 1950s*, Basingstoke: Palgrave Macmillan.

Field, Clive (2017) *Secularization in the Long 1960s: Numerating Religion in Britain*, Oxford: Oxford University Press.

Field, Clive (2019) *Periodizing Secularization: Religious Allegiance and Attendance in Britain, 1880–1945*, Oxford: Oxford University Press.

Field, Clive (2021) *Counting Religion in Britain, 1970–2020*, Oxford: Oxford University Press.

File on 4 (2022) 'Modern slavery in the care sector', BBC Radio 4, 25 July. www.bbc.co.uk/programmes/m001p1tl

Financial Times (2023) 'Care conundrum: demographic shifts create jobs but not workers'. https://www.ft.com/content/e624b426-3ac0-426d-b6a4-40e52333e51b

Finlayson, Lorna (2022) 'Door close, backs turn', *London Review of Books*, 44(9): 25–7.

Fleming, Mick (2023) *Blown Away: From Drug Dealer to Life Bringer*, London: SPCK.

Foster, Alicia (2023) *Gwen John: Art and Life in London and Paris*, London: Thames and Hudson.

Fraser, Giles (2018) 'How the Church lost its flock over Brexit', *UnHerd*, 23 November. www.unherd.com/2018/11/church-lost-flock-brexit

Freathy, Rob, and Parker, Stephen G. (2013) 'Secularists, humanists and religious education: religious crisis and curriculum change in England 1963–75', *History of Education*, 42(2): 22–56.

Funder, Anna (2023) *Wifedom: Mrs Orwell's Invisible Life*, London: Viking.

Garvey, Jane, and Bere, Jemma (2022) 'A phone call changed my life forever', *Life Changing*, BBC Radio 4. www.bbc.co.uk/programmes/articles/1nSV0Rn2zJQqyvNs2Tz2XjH/a-phone-call-changed-my-life-forever

Gavron, Hannah (1966) *The Captive Wife: Conflicts of Housebound Mothers*, London: Routledge and Kegan Paul.

Gill, Martha (2023) 'To those who claim the NHS has turned into a British religion, I say: keep the faith', *The Guardian*, 9 July. www.theguardian.com/commentisfree/2023/jul/09/nhs-british-religion-keep-faith-nhs-at-75

Gilligan, Carol (1982) *In a Different Voice: Psychological Theory and Women's Development*, Cambridge, MA: Harvard University Press.

Gilligan, Carol (2023) *In a Human Voice*, Cambridge: Polity.

Gilmore, Maeve (1970) *A World Away: A Memoir of Mervyn Peake*, London: Gollancz.

Goldman, Ronald J. (1965) 'Do we want our children taught about God?', *New Society*, 27 May, pp 8–10.

Goodhart, David (2017) *The Road to Somewhere: The Populist Revolt and the Future of Politics*, London: Hurst.

Goodhart, David (2020) *Head, Hand, Heart: The Struggle for Dignity and Status in the 21st Century*, London: Allen Lane.

Government Statistics on Corona Virus and Home Schooling (2021); www.ons.gov.uk/peoplepopulationandcommunity/educationandchildcare/articles/coronavirusandhomeschooling

Gray, Susan (2023) 'Television', *The Church Times*, 3 November, p 30.

Greer, Germaine (1970) *The Female Eunuch*, London: McGibbon and Kee.

Griffin, Emma (2020) *Bread Winner: An Intimate History of the Victorian Economy*, New Haven, CT: Yale University Press.

Guest, Mathew (2017) 'From Jevons to Collini (via Douglas Davies): reflections on higher education and religious identity', in Guest, Mathew, with Middlemiss Le-Bon, M. (eds) *Death, Life and Laughter: Essays on Religion in Honour of Douglas Davies*, London: Routledge, pp 201–20.

Guest, Mathew (2022) *Neoliberal Religion: Faith and Power in the Twenty-First Century*, London: Bloomsbury.

Guest, Mathew, and Aune, Kristin (2017) 'Students' construction of a Christiam future: faith, class and aspiration in university contexts', *Sociological Research Online*, 22(1): art 12. http://socresonline.org.uk/22/1/12.html

Hare, Brian, and Woods, Vanessa (2020) *Survival of the Friendliest: Understanding our Origins and Rediscovering our Common Humanity*, London: Penguin.

Harrington, Mary (2023) *Feminism against Progress*, Croydon: Forum.

Hatcher, Mark (2023) *Bishops in the House of Lords: Fit for the Future?* LLM Dissertation in Canon Law, Cardiff University.

Health Foundation (2023) *Health in 2040*. www.health.org.uk/publications/health-in-2040

Hennessy, Peter (2022) *A Duty of Care: Britain Before and After Covid*, London: Penguin.

Herbert, George (1633/2017) 'The elixir', in *The Temple* (Reprint), London: Penguin, pp 291–2.

HESA (2024) 'Higher Education Student Statistics: UK, 2022/23 - Student numbers and characteristics'. https://researchbriefings.files.parliament.uk/documents/CBP-7857/CBP-7857.pdf

Higgins, Charlotte (2016) 'Is opera the most misogynistic art form?', *The Guardian*, 26 February. www.theguardian.com/music/2016/feb/26/is-opera-the-most-misogynistic-art-form

Hochschild, Arlie, with Machung, Anne (1989) *The Second Shift: Working Parents and the Revolution at Home*, New York: Viking.

Hocking, Silas K. (nd) *Her Benny*, London: Frederick Warne.

Hogan, Anne, and Bradstock, Andrew (eds) (1998) *Women of Faith in Victorian Culture: Reassessing 'the Angel in the House'*, Basingstoke: Palgrave Macmillan.

House of Commons Library (2023) 'Delayed hospital discharges and adult social care'. https://commonslibrary.parliament.uk/delayed-hospital-discharges-and-adult-social-care/#:~:textOn%209%20January%202023%20

Independent Inquiry into Child Sexual Abuse (2019) 'The Anglican Church investigation report'. www.iicsa.org.uk/reports-recommendations/publications/investigation/anglican-church/executive-summary.html

Independent Inquiry into Child Sexual Abuse (2020) 'The Roman Catholic Church investigation report'. www.iicsa.org.uk/reports-recommendations/publications/investigation/roman-catholic-church#:~The%20Independent%20Inquiry%20into%20Child%20Sexual%20Abuse

Institute for Fiscal Studies (2021) *Inequalities in Education, Skills and Incomes in the UK: Implications of the Covid-19 Pandemic*. https://ifs.org.uk/publications/inequalities-education-skills-and-incomes-uk-implications-covid-19-pandemic

Institute for Fiscal Studies (2023) *Implications of the NHS Workforce Plan.* https://ifs.org.uk/publications/implications-nhs-workforce-plan

Ishiguro, Katsuo (2005) *Never Let Me Go*, London: Faber.

Ishiguro, Katsuo (2021) *Klara and the Sun*, London: Faber.

Jacobson, Howard (2022) *Mother's Boy: A Writer's Beginnings*, London: Jonathan Cape.

Jeffreys, Branwen (2022) 'Covid pandemic fuels deepening education inequalities in England, say MPs', *BBC News*, 11 March. www.bbc.co.uk/news/education-60683839

Johnson, Alan (2018) *In My Life: A Music Memoir*, London: Penguin.

Johnson, Paul (2023) *Follow the Money: How Much Does Britain Cost?* London: Little Brown.

Jolly, Margaretta (2019) *Sisterhood and After: An Oral History of the UK Women's Liberation Movement, 1968-Present*, Oxford: Oxford University Press.

Jones, Lee (2019) 'The seven deadly sins of marketisation in British higher education', *Bella Caledonia*, 4 December. www.bellacaledonia.org.uk/2019/12/04/the-seven-deadly-sins-of-marketisation-in-british-higher-education

Jones, Timothy Willem (2013) *Sexual Politics in the Church of England, 1857–1957*, Oxford, Oxford University Press.

Katz, Roberta, Ogilvie, Sarah, Shaw, Jane, and Woodhead, Linda (eds) (2021) *Gen Z Explained: The Art of Living in a Digital Age*, Chicago, IL: University of Chicago Press.

Keating, Jenny (nd) *Adoption in England and Wales: The Twentieth Century*. www.historyandpolicy.org/docs/dfe-jenny-keating.pdf

Kenway, Emily (2023) *Who Cares: The Hidden Crisis of Caregiving and How We Solve It*, London: Headline.

Kernan, Joseph (2006) 'Verdi and the undoing of women', *Cambridge Opera Journal*, 18(1): 21–31.

Khalili, Laleh (2023) 'Woke capital', *London Review of Books*, 45(17): 20–1.

Kittay, Eva Feder (2002) 'When caring is just and justice is caring: justice and mental retardation', in Kittay, Eva Feder, and Feder, Ellen K. (eds) *The Subject of Care: Feminist Perspectives on Dependency*, London: Rowman and Littlefield, pp 257–76.

Klein, Stephan (2014) *The Survival of the Nicest: How Altruism Made us Human and How it Pays to Get Along* (Trans Dollenmayer, David), Brunswick: Scribe.

Kolpinskaya, Ekaterina, and Fox, Stuart (2021) *Religion and Euroscepticism in Brexit Britain*, Abingdon: Routledge.

Koram, Koko (2022) *Uncommon Wealth: Britain and the Aftermath of Empire*, London: John Murray.

Koram, Koko (2023) 'Hail, hail, Freedonia!', *Times Literary Supplement*, 6273: 11–12.

Kumar, Krishan (2021) *A Historical and Political Sociology*, Cambridge: Polity.

Kynaston, David (2021) 'Better all the time: the complicated relation between education and equality', *Times Literary Supplement*, 26 February, p 12.

Lang, Marjory (1980) 'Childhood's champions: mid-Victorian's periodicals and the critics', *Victorian Periodicals Review*, 13: 17–21.

Lawson, Dominic (2023) 'My father was right about the NHS being a national religion – but now striking medics are abusing our faith', *The Daily Mail*, 17 April. www.dailymail.co.uk/debate/article-11979789-DOMINIC-LAWSON-father-right-nhs-national-religion

Lee, Hermione (2007) *Virginia Woolf*, London: Chatto and Windus.

Light, Alison (2008) *Mrs Woolf and the Servants*, London Penguin.

Light, Alison (2019) *A Radical Romance: A Memoir of Love, Grief and Consolation*, London: Penguin.

Light, Alison (2020) 'Behind the green baize door', *London Review of Books*, 42(2): 21.

Light, Alison (2022) *Inside History: From Popular Poets to Life Writing*, Edinburgh: Edinburgh University Press.

Lockwood, Patricia (2021) '"Pull off my head" (Review of *Bear* by Marian Engel)', *London Review of Books*, 23(16): 7–10.

Lomax, Elaine (2008) 'Telling the other side: Hesba Stretton's "Outcast" stories', in Briggs, Julia, Potts, Dennis, and Orville-Grenville, Matthew (eds) *Popular Children's Literature*, Farnham: Ashgate, pp 143–8.

Lomax, Elaine (2009) *The Writings of Hesba Stretton: Reclaiming the Outcast*, Aldershot: Ashgate.

Maby, Tim (2020) 'Is the NHS our new national religion?', *Religion Media Centre*, 14 April. https://religionmediacentre.org.uk/news/is-the-nhs-our-new-national-religion/

Macnicol, John (2015) *Neoliberalising Old Age*, Cambridge: Cambridge University Press.

Maguire, David, Honeyman, Matthew, Fenny, Deborah, and Jabba, Joni (2021) *Shaping the Future of Digital Technology in Health and Social Care*, The King's Fund. https://assets.kingsfund.org.uk/f/256914/x/f6444844fd/shaping_future_digital_technology_health_social_care_2021.pdf

Malik, Kenan (2020) 'The rise of white identity politics', *Prospect Magazine*, 13 July.

Malik, Kenan (2023) *Not So Black and White: A History of Race from White Supremacy to Identity Politics*, London: Hurst.

Malone, Michael (1984) *Handling Sin*, Boston, MA: Little Brown & Co.

Mandler, Peter (2020) *The Crisis of the Meritocracy: Britain's Transition to Mass Education since the Second World War*, Oxford: Oxford University Press.

Marmot, M. (2010) *Fair Society, Healthy Lives: The Marmot Review*. www.gov.uk/research-for-development-outputs/fair-society-healthy-lives-the-marmot-review-strategic-review-of-health-inequalities-in-england-post-2010

Marmot, Michael, Allen, Jessica, Boyce, Tammy, Goldblatt, Peter, Morrison, Joana (2020) *Health Equity in England: The Marmot Review Ten Years on*, London: Institute of Health Equity. www.instituteofhealthequity.org/resources-reports/marmot-review-10-years-on

Marmot, Michael and Bambra, Clare (2023) 'Evidence to Covid-19 Inquiry', *BBC News*, 16 June.

Martin, Bernice (1981) *A Sociology of Contemporary Cultural Change*, Oxford: Blackwell.

Martin, Bernice (1984) '"Mother wouldn't like it!" Housework as magic', *Theory, Culture and Society*, 2(2): 19–36.

Martin, Bernice (2001) 'The Pentecostal gender paradox', in Fenn, R.K. (ed) *The Blackwell Companion to Sociology of Religion*, Oxford: Blackwell, pp 52–66.

Martin, Bernice (2013) 'Tensions and trends in Pentecostal gender and family relations', in Heffner, Robert W. (ed) *Global Pentecostalism in the 21st Century*, Bloomington: Indiana University Press, pp 115–48.

Martin, David (1967) *A Sociology of English Religion*, London: SCM.

Martin, David (2018) 'Thinking with your life', in Hans, Joas (ed) *David Martin and the Sociology of Religion*, Abingdon: Routledge, pp 162–208.

Martin, Jessica (2019) 'Dorothy L. Sayers (1893–1957): God and the detective', in Maltby, Judith, and Shell, Alison (eds) *Anglican Women Novelists: From Charlotte Bronte to P.D. James*, London: T&T Clark, pp 86–101.

Martin, Jessica (2020) *Holiness and Desire*, London: Canterbury Press.

Martin, Jessica (2023) *The Eucharist in Four Dimensions* (The Bampton Lectures 2021), Norwich: Canterbury.

Mazzucato, Mariana (2019) *The Value of Everything: Making and Taking in the Global Economy*, London: Penguin.

Mazzucato, Mariana (2022) *Mission Economy: A Moonshot Guide to Changing Capitalism*, London: Penguin.

McCrindle, Jean, and Rowbotham, Sheila (eds) (1977) *Dutiful Daughters: Women Talk about their Lives*, London: Allen Lane.

McLeod, Hugh (2005) 'The religious crisis of the 1960s', *Journal of Modern European History*, 3(2): 205–30.

McLeod, Hugh (2007) *The Religious Crisis of the 1960s*, Oxford: Oxford University Press.

McLeod, Hugh (2013) 'Reflections and new perspectives', in Christie, Nancy, and Gavreau, Michael (eds) *The Sixties and Beyond: Dechristianization in Western Europe and North America*, Toronto: University of Toronto Press, pp 453–68.

McLeod, Hugh (2022) *Religion and the Rise of Sport in England*, Oxford: Oxford University Press.

McNaught, Matthew (2022) *Immanuel*, London: Fitzcarraldo.

Millett, Kate (1970) *Sexual Politics*, New York: Doubleday.

Moran, Caitlin (2022) 'Interview with the Rev. Richard Coles', *The Times Magazine*, 26 May, pp 24–9.

Moran, Joe (2023) 'Gen Z and me', *London Review of Books*, 45(4): 20–1.

Moyse, Cordelia (2009) *A History of the Mothers' Union: Women, Anglicanism and Globalisation, 1976–2008*, Woodbridge: Boydell.

Munt, Sally (1994) *Murder by the Book: Feminism and the Crime Novel*, London: Routledge.

National Churches Trust (2020) *House of Good: The Economic and Social Value of Church Buildings to the UK*, London: National Churches Trust. www.houseofgood.nationalchurchestrust.org/wp-content/uploads/2020/10/House-of-Good-AW-digital-small.pdf

NHS England (2023) *NHS Long Term Workforce Plan.* www.england.nhs.uk/long-read/nhs-long-term-workforce-plan-2/

Oakley, Ann (1974) *The Sociology of Housework*, London: Martin Robertson.

Oakley, Ann (2019) *The Sociology of Housework* (reissue with a new introduction), Bristol: Policy Press.

Oakley, Ann (2021) *Forgotten Wives: How Women Get Written out of History*, Bristol: Policy Press.

O'Driscoll, Sean (2022) *Heiress, Rebel, Vigilante, Bomber: The Extraordinary Life of Rose Dugdale*, Dublin: Sandycove.

Office for National Statistics (2015) 'How religion has changed in England and Wales', 4 June. www.ons.gov.uk/peoplepopulationandcommunity/culturalidentity/religion/articles/howreligionhaschangedinenglandandwales/2015-06-04

Office for National Statistics (2021) 'Corona virus and home schooling'. www.ons.gov.uk/peoplepopulationandcommunity/educationandchildcare/articles/coronavirusandhomeschooling

Office for National Statistics (2022a) 'Ethnic group, England and Wales: Census 2021', 29 November. www.ons.gov.uk/peoplepopulationandcommunity/culturalidentity/ethnicity/bulletins/ethnicgroupenglandandwales/census2021

Office for National Statistics (2022b) 'Religion, England and Wales: Census 2021', 29 November. www.ons.gov.uk/peoplepopulationandcommunity/culturalidentity/religion/bulletins/religionenglandandwales/census2021

Office for National Statistics (2023) 'Unpaid care by age, sex and deprivation, England and Wales: Census 2021'. www.ons.gov.uk/peoplepopulationandcommunity/healthandsocialcare/socialcare/articles/unpaidcarebyagesexanddeprivationenglandandwales/census2021

Ofsted (2021) 'Review of Sexual Abuse in Schools and Colleges', GOV.UK. www.gov.uk/government/publications/review-of-sexual-abuse-in-schools-and-colleges

Olusoga, David (2023) *Our NHS: A Hidden History*, documentary. www.bbc.co.uk/programmes/m000xwz6

Orr, Deborah (2020) *Motherwell: A Girlhood*, London: Weidenfeld and Nicolson.

Paley, Chris (2021) *Beyond Bad: How Obsolete Morals are Holding Us Back*, London: Coronet.

Parvez, Anam (2023) *Radical Pathways beyond GDP*, Oxfam Discussion Paper. https://oxfamilibrary.openrepository.com/bitstream/handle/10546/621532/dp-radical-pathways-beyond-gdp-03082023-en.pdf;jsessionid=BF8548596D694B5E627D72817F0696BB?sequence=4

Peake, Christian (nd) 'maeve_gilmore_archive', *Instagram.* www.instagram.com/maeve_gilmore_archive

Perrin, Ruth (2020) *Changing Shape: The Faith Lives of Millennials*, London: SCM.

Perry, Louise (2022) *The Case Against the Sexual Revolution*, Cambridge: Polity.

Piesse, Jude (2021) *The Ghost in the Garden: In Search of Darwin's Lost Garden*, London: Scribe.

Piketty, Thomas (2013) *Capital in the Twenty-First Century*, Cambridge, MA: Harvard University Press.

Raihani, Nichola (2021) *The Social Instinct: How Cooperation Shaped the World*, London: Jonathan Cape.

Rajan, Amol (2023) 'Rethink work' *Jobs of the Future*, No 3, BBC Radio 4 discussion panel conducted by Amol Rajan with David Goodhart and others, 3 August.

Reynolds, Kimberley (2008) 'Rewarding reads? Giving, receiving and resisting Evangelical rewards and prize books', in Briggs, Julia, Potts, Dennis, and Orville-Grenby, Matthew (eds) *Popular Children's Literature in Britain*, Farnham: Ashgate, pp 189–208.

Robbins, Joel (2004) 'The globalisation of Pentecostal and charismatic Christianity', *Annual Review of Anthropology*, 3: 117–43.

Roberts, Elizabeth (1995) *Women and Families: An Oral History, 1940–1970*, Oxford: Blackwell.

Robinson, John (1963) *Honest to God*, London: SCM.

Roe, Dinah (2022) 'Tale of Tender Lizzie: the centrality of caring in Christina Rossetti's work', *Times Literary Supplement*, 6219, 10 September, p 13.

Rowbotham, Sheila (2021) *Daring to Hope: My Life in the 1970s*, London and New York: Verso.

Roy, Olivier (2019) *Is Europe Christian?* Oxford: Oxford University Press.

Roy, Olivier (2020) 'Is Europe Christian?', *The Immanent Frame*. https://tif.ssrc.org/category/book-blog/book-forums/is-europe-christian/?

Runciman, David (2023) *The Handover: How We Gave Control of Our Lives to Corporations, States and AIs*, London: Profile.

Russell, Stuart (2020) *Human Compatible: AI and the Problem of Control*, London: Penguin.

Russell, Stuart (2021) The Reith Lectures on 'Living with Artificial Intelligence', BBC Radio 4. www.bbc.co.uk/programmes/m001216k

Ryrie, Alec (2019) *Unbelievers: An Emotional History of Doubt*, Cambridge, MA: Harvard University Press.

Sampson, Fiona (2021) *Two Way Mirror: The Life of Elizabeth Barratt Browning*, London: Profile.

Samuel, Mithran (2023) 'Staff abused women at learning disability unit, finds CQC', *Community Care*, 23 September. www.communitycare.co.uk/2020/09/23/staff-abused-women-learning-disability-unit-finds-cqc

Savage, Mike (2021) *The Return of Inequality: Social Change and the Weight of the Past*, Cambridge, MA: Harvard University Press.

Schuezte, Christy K. (2023) *Spirit Wives and Church Mothers: Marriage, Survival and Healing in Central Mozambique*, Maddison: University of Wisconsin Press.

Schwartz, Laura (2019) *Feminism and the Servant Problem: Class and Domestic Labour in the Women's Suffrage Movement*, Cambridge: Cambridge University Press.

Scott, Joan Wallach (2018) *Sex and Secularism*: Princeton, NJ: Princeton University Press.

Seaton, Andrew (2023) *Our NHS: A History of London's Best-Loved Institution*, New Haven, CT: Yale University Press.

Seligman, Adam (2000) *Modernity's Wager: Authority, the Self, and Transcendence*, Princeton, NJ: Princeton University Press.

Shafik, Minouche (2021) *What We Owe Each Other: A New Social Contract*, London: Bodley Head.

Sissay, Lemn (2017) *Gold From the Stone*, Edinburgh: Canongate.

Sissay, Lemn (2019) *My Name is Why: A Memoir*, Edinburgh: Canongate.

Sissay, Lemn (2023) *Let the Light Pour In: Morning Poems*, Edinburgh: Canongate.

Sixsmith, Martin (2009) *The Lost Child of Philomena Lee*, London: Macmillan.

Skills for Care (2022) *The State of the Adult Social Care Sector and Workforce in England*. Leeds: Skills for Care. www.skillsforcare.org.uk/Adult=Social-Care-Workforce-Data/Workforce-intelligence/publications/national-information

Slobodian, Quinn (2023) *Crack-Up Capitalism: Market Radicals and the Dream of a World without Democracy*, London: Allen Lane.

Smith, Christian, and Adamczyk, Amy (2021) *Handing on the Faith: How Parents Pass their Religion on to the Next Generation*, Oxford: Oxford University Press.

Sobolewska, Maria, and Ford, Robert (2020) *Brexitland: Identity, Diversity and the Reshaping of British Politics*, Cambridge: Cambridge University Press.

Spalding, Frances (2022) *The Real and the Romantic: English Art between the Wars*, London: Thames and Hudson.

Spencer, Nick (2016) *Doing Good: A Future for Faith in the Public Square*, London: Theos. www.theosthinktank.co.uk/cmsfiles/archive/files/Reports/TheosBookletfinal.pdf

Spufford, Margaret (1989) *Celebration: A Story of Suffering and Joy*, London: Mobray.

Steedman, Carolyn (1986) *Landscape for a Good Woman*, London: Virago.

Steedman, Carolyn (2009) *Labours Lost: Domestic Service and the Making of Modern* England, Cambridge: Cambridge University Press.

Stewart, John (2020) *Richard Titmuss: A Commitment to Welfare*, Bristol: Bristol University Press/Policy Press. https://doi.org/10.2307/j.ctv 128f qbs

Stewart, Rory (2023) *Politics on the Edge: A Memoir from Within*, London: Jonathan Cape.

St Martin in the Fields (2023) 'Autumn lecture series 2023 – Here I stand, I can do no other', 16 October. http://www.stmartin-in-the-fields.org/congregational-life/lecture-series-2023/#:~:text=2023%E2%80%99s%20St%20Martin-in-the-Fields%20Autumn%20Lectures

Storey, David (2021) *A Stinging Delight*, London: Faber.

Stretton, Hesba (Undated) (1865) *Jessica's First Prayer*, London: The Religious Tract Society (originally in *Sunday at Home*, 1866).

Stretton, Hesba (Undated) (1868) *Little Meg's Children*, London: The Religious Tract Society (reprinted Minneapolis MN: Curiosmith, 2010).

Stretton, Hesba (Undated) (1904) *Jessica's Mother*, London: The Religious Tract Society (originally in *Sunday at Home* 1866).

Strhan, Anna, and Shillitoe, Rachael (2019) 'The stickiness of non-religion? Intergenerational transition and the formation of non-religious identities in childhood', *Sociology*, 53(6): 1094–110.

Strhan, Anna, and Shillitoe, Rachael (2022) 'The experience of non-religious children in religious education', *Journal of Religious Education*. doi 10.1007/s40839-022-00180-y

Stringer, Martin (1999) *On the Perception of Worship in Three Christian Congregations in Manchester*, Birmingham: Birmingham University Press.

Stringer, Martin (2008) *Contemporary Western Ethnography and the Definition of Religion*, London: Continuum.

Stuart, Douglas (2020) *Shuggie Bain*, London: Picador.

Suleyman, Mustafa, and Bhaksar, Michael (2023) *The Coming Wave: Technology, Power and the Twenty-First Century's Greatest Dilemma*, London: Vintage.

Susina, Jan (2009) *The Place of Lewis Carroll in Children's Literature*, New York: Routledge.

Susskind, Daniel (2020) *A World without Work: Innovation and How We Should Respond*, London: Allen Lane.

Sylvester, Rachel (2023) 'How Japan is solving its age problem: would it work in the UK?' *Times Magazine*, 12 August, pp 42–7.

Taylor, Catherine (2021) '"Triumph and disaster" (Review of David Storey's memoir)', *Times Literary Supplement*, 6168.

Taylor, Charles (1989) *Sources of the Self: The Making of the Modern Identity*, Cambridge, MA: Harvard University Press.

Taylor, Charles (1999) 'A Catholic modernity?', in Heft, James L. (ed) *Charles Taylor's Marianist Award Lecture for 1996*, Oxford: Oxford University Press, pp 13–37.

Taylor, Charles (2003) *Modern Social Imaginaries*, Durham, NC: Duke University Press.

Taylor, Charles (2007) *A Secular Age*, Cambridge, MA: Harvard University Press.

Taylor, Ros (2018) 'How Anglicans tipped the Brexit vote', *LSE*, 20 September. https://blogs.lse.ac.uk/brexit/2018/09/20/how-anglicans-tipped-the-brexit-vote/

Thane, Pat, and Evans, Tanya (2012) *Sinners? Scroungers? Saints? Unmarried Motherhood in Twentieth-Century England*, Oxford: Oxford University Press.

The Guardian (2022) 'The Guardian view on Maeve Gilmore's art: out from the shadows', 15 May. www.theguardian.com/commentisfree/2022/may/15/the-guardian-view-on-maeve-gilmores-art-out-from-the-shadows

Thomas, Ed (2020) 'Burnley's Pastor Mick – from dangerous drug dealer to lifesaver', *BBC News*, 18 December. www.bbc.co.uk/news/stories-55273677

Thompson, Naomi (2017) *Young People and Church since 1900: Engagement and Exclusion*, London: Routledge.

Thurman, Neil, Cornia, Alessio, and Kunert, Jessica (2016) *Journalists in the UK*, Reuters Institute for the Study of Journalism. https://reutersinstitute.politics.ox.ac.uk/our-research/journalists-uk

Todd, Selina (2020) *Snakes and Ladders: The Great Social Mobility Myth*, London: Chatto and Windus.

Tomalin, Claire (2012) *The Invisible Woman: The Story of Nelly Ternan and Charles Dickens*, London: Penguin.

Topp, Sylvia (2021) *Eileen: The Making of George Orwell*, London: Unbound.

Toynbee, Polly (2018) 'The NHS is our religion: it's the only thing that saves it from the Tories', *The Guardian*, 3 July. www.theguardian.com/commentisfree/2018/jul/03/nhs-religion-tories-health-service

Voigt, Gabriel, and König, Anne-Sophie L. (2021) 'Robotic devices and ICT in long-term care in Japan: their potential and limitations from a workplace perspective', *Contemporary Japan*. doi: 10.1080/18692729.2021.2015846

Wade, Francesca (2020) *Square Haunting: Five Women, Freedom and London between the Wars*, London: Faber.

Wade, Francesca (2022) 'At Studio Voltaire', *London Review of Books*, 44 (13): 33.

Wagner, Anne M. (2013) 'Lowry, repetition and change', in Clark, J.T. and Wagner, Anne M. (eds) *Lowry and the Painting of Modern Life* (Exhibition catalogue), London: Tate Publishing, pp 75–122.

Walsh, Tony (2013) *Sex & Love & Rock&Roll*, Portishead: Burning Eye Books.

Wanless, Derek (2002) Securing our Future Health: Taking a Long-Term View, The King's Fund. www.yearofcare.co.uk/sites/default/files/images/Wanless.pdf

Ward, Stuart (2023) *United Kingdom: A Global History of the End of Britain*, Cambridge: Cambridge University Press.

White, Hannah (2022) *The Nones: Who Are They and What do They Believe?* London: Theos. www.theosthinktank.co.uk/research/2022/10/31/the-nones-who-are-they-and-what-do-they-believe

Williams, Roderick (2020) 'Courtesans and captains', *Britain in Ten Operas*, Radio 4. www.bbc.co.uk/programmes/m000pghg

Williams, Rowan (2022) 'Freedom of worship', The Reith Lectures on 'The Four Freedoms', Lecture 2, BBC Radio 4. www.bbc.co.uk/sounds/play/m001fw1l

Willing, Nick (2017) *Paula Rego: Secrets and Stories*, Documentary, BBC Four, 23 March.

Wills, Clare (2021) 'Architectures of confinement', *London Review of Books*, 43(10): 17–22.

Wills, Clare (2023) *The Family Plot: Three Pieces about Containment*, London: LRB Books.

Wincer, Penny (2020) *Tender: The Imperfect Art of Caring*, London: Coronet.

Woodhead, Linda (2012) 'Introduction', in Woodhead, L. and Catto, Rebecca (eds) *Religion and Change in Modern Britain*, London: Routledge, pp 10–33.

Woodhead, Linda (2020) 'The NHS, our national religion', *Religion Media Centre*, 1 April. www.religiousmediacentre.org.uk/news/the-nhs-our-national-religion/2/03/2020

Woodhead, Linda (2021) *Values Are the New Religion*, Cadbury Lectures. www.birmingham.ac.uk/schools/ptr/departments/theologyandreligion/events/cadburylectures/2021

Woodhead, Linda, and Catto, Rebecca (eds) (2012) *Religion and Change in Modern Britain*, London: Routledge.

Wooldridge, Adrian (2021) *The Aristocracy of Talent: How Meritocracy Made the Modern World*, London: Allen Lane.

Woolf, Virginia (1935) *A Room of One's Own*, London: Hogarth.

Woolf, Virginia (1938) *Three Guineas*, London: Hogarth.

World Economic Forum (2019) 'Japan's workforce will be 20% smaller by 2040', 12 February. www.weforum.org/agenda/2019/02/japan-s-workforce-will-shrink-20-by-2040

Young, Frances (2014) *Arthur's Call*, London: SPCK.

Zuboff, Shoshana (2019) *The Age of Surveillance Capitalism: The Fight for a Human Future and the Frontier of Power*, London: Profile.

Index

References to endnotes show both the page number and the note number (173n2).

T

U

V

W

Printed and bound by CPI Group (UK) Ltd, Croydon, CR0 4YY
15/09/2026
14962388-0002